SeaWise

SAFETY CHECKLIST

FOR MOTOR YACHTS

Off-Shore Voyage Preparation

Engine Diagram

Safety Briefing

Deck Plan

Critical Immediate-Access Equipment

Stow Plan

On Watch

Fuel Consumption

Heavy Weather Preparation

Kits

Specs & Limitations

Equipment Lists

Created By Zvi Richard Dor-Ner & Zvi Frank

CMP

Overwrap Photo: Speed boat in tropical sea
© Iakov Kalinin. Courtesy of Bigstockphoto.com.

Library of Congress Control Number: 2015930250

Type set in Akzidenz Grotesk

ISBN: 978-0-87033-639-3

Printed in China

Published by Schiffer Publishing, Ltd.
4880 Lower Valley Road
Atglen, PA 19310
Phone: (610) 593-1777; Fax: (610) 593-2002
E-mail: Info@schifferbooks.com

For our complete selection of fine books on this and related subjects, please visit our website at www.schifferbooks.com. You may also write for a free catalog.

This book may be purchased from the publisher. Please try your bookstore first.

We are always looking for people to write books on new and related subjects. If you have an idea for a book, please contact us at proposals@schifferbooks.com.

Schiffer Publishing's titles are available at special discounts for bulk purchases for sales promotions or premiums. Special editions, including personalized covers, corporate imprints, and excerpts can be created in large quantities for special needs. For more information, contact the publisher.

US $50.00
9 780870 336393 55000
ISBN: 978-0-87033-639-3

1

1. Off-Shore Voyage Preparation

1. NAVIGATION

- ❒ Check and mark paper charts and plotter.
- ❒ Annotate pilot books and tide tables.
- ❒ Mark course and distance.
- ❒ Scrutinize course for obstacles, shallows, and landmarks.
- ❒ Note alternate harbors and shelters.

2. COMMUNICATIONS

- ❒ Identify SAR and medical assistance frequencies and contact numbers for mobile and satellite phone for the area where you are sailing.
- ❒ Identify radio channels for harbors and shore stations along the course.
- ❒ Identify time and frequencies of weather broadcasts on VHF and SSB.
- ❒ Secure a land-based advocate—a friend who knows you and your plans and, if necessary, can represent your interests to the authorities.
- ❒ File sailing plans with your advocate.

3. WEATHER

- ❒ Follow weather patterns days before departure.
- ❒ Get the pilot charts' statistics for the time period.
- ❒ Identify weather sources on the Internet.
- ❒ Identify general (GRIB) and local (Coast Guard) sources for forecasts.

Continued On Next Page

4. CREW

- ❐ Have the right crew for the voyage, taking into account sea conditions, weather, and passage length; favor crew with specific skills, medical or mechanical.
- ❐ Crew susceptible to seasickness should not drink alcohol for twenty-four hours before departure and should start seasickness medication at that time.
- ❐ Do not allow alcohol or drugs on board during a passage.
- ❐ Perform a safety crew briefing.

  See 2. Safety Briefing, p. 5. ***(Safety Checklist)***
- ❐ Review and confirm accessibility to Critical Equipment.

  See 3. Critical Immediate-Access Equipment, p. 7. ***(Safety Checklist)***

5. INSPECTIONS

- ❐ Check engine oil, gear oil, and water.
- ❐ Make sure the alternator is charging.
- ❐ Check that all instruments are working.
- ❐ Inspect the rig for integrity.
- ❐ Check steering system.
- ❐ Have a plan and the necessary fittings on board to construct a makeshift rudder.
- ❐ Have a hole drilled in the upper, outer part of the rudder, capable of taking a line.
- ❐ Have the emergency tiller ready and accessible.
- ❐ Check engine gears and thruster.
- ❐ Check radio equipment.

6. PROVISIONING

- ❐ Top off water and diesel; have spare engine fluids and filters.
- ❐ Have ample food for length of passage and size of crew.
- ❐ Prepare meals for the first 24 hours, and stock provisions necessary to prepare several days' worth of oven-ready, one-pot meals.
- ❐ Provide sweets and snacks for night watches.
- ❐ Fill thermoses with hot water for soups and hot drinks.
- ❐ Empty holding tanks.

2. Safety Briefing

The safety briefing is to acquaint the crew with the safety procedures of the boat and to assess the abilities and limitations of the crew.

The skipper should should obtain and review all personal and medical information about the crew that could have an impact on the safe operation of the boat.

2

1. GOVERNANCE

There is precise governance on a boat. There is only one captain, and the safety briefing is the right place to establish this. Identify mates, watch leaders, and so on.

See 13. Skipper Disabled, p. 91. ***(Action Guide)***

2. CREW ABILITIES AND CARE

- ❒ Relevant experience
- ❒ Medical conditions and medications
- ❒ Swimming ability
- ❒ Seasickness medication experience
- ❒ Sun exposure

3. SAFETY IN COCKPIT AND ON DECK

- ❒ Never go on deck without another crew member in the cockpit.
- ❒ Non-swimmers should never leave the cockpit without a life vest.
- ❒ Enforce life vest and harness policy in heavy weather and at night.
- ❒ Demonstrate safe operation of winches, autopilot, steering wheel, and engine.
- ❒ Demonstrate deck line and fender handling.

Continued On Next Page

4. MAN OVERBOARD

- ❐ Review and summarize procedures.

  See 9. Man Overboard, p. 67. ***(Action Guide)***

5. FIRE

- ❐ Leave no fire unattended, e.g., stove, lights, BBQ, etc.
- ❐ Establish smoking policy.
- ❐ Identify location of all firefighting equipment.

  See 3. Critical Immediate-Access Equipment, p. 7. ***(Safety Checklist)***

6. EMERGENCY COMMUNICATION

- ❐ Demonstrate basic operation of radios and telephone.
- ❐ Review message format and content

  See 7. Emergency Communications, p. 37. ***(Action Guide)***

7. SKIPPER INCAPACITATED

- ❐ Review procedures.

  See 13. Skipper Disabled, p. 91. ***(Action Guide)***

  Note: Remind the crew, when in doubt, ask!

3. Critical Immediate-Access Equipment

All crew members should know the location of critical equipment and fittings. These items should be readily available when needed, and the crew should know how to use them.
See 9. Stow Plan, p. 29. ***(Safety Checklist)***

1. PERSONAL

- ❐ Life vests
- ❐ Flashlight
- ❐ Knife
- ❐ MOB rig and strobe
- ❐ Lifesling
- ❐ First aid kit

3

2. FIRE

- ❐ Fire extinguishers
- ❐ Fire blanket
- ❐ Hoses and buckets
- ❐ Fuel shut-off
- ❐ Propane cylinder shut-off

3. WATER

- ❐ Bilge alarm and bilge pump switch
- ❐ Manual pump
- ❐ Buckets
- ❐ Seacocks and plugs

Continued On Next Page

4. DAMAGE CONTROL

- ❒ Emergency tiller
- ❒ Fenders and mooring lines
- ❒ Working tools
- ❒ Damage control kit

5. RESCUE

- ❒ EPIRB
- ❒ Handheld VHF
- ❒ Mobile and satellite phones
- ❒ Ditch bag
- ❒ Life raft
- ❒ Dinghy
- ❒ Pyrotechnics

See 9. Stow Plan, p. 29. ***(Safety Checklist)***

4. On Watch

The crew member on watch has complete responsibility for the welfare of the vessel and the crew. On watch, the crew member is in charge of boat operations and safety.

WATCH HANDOFF

- ❐ Course and speed to maintain
- ❐ Traffic in the vicinity
- ❐ Ground landmarks and markers
- ❐ Wind and sea status and forecast
- ❐ Engine status
- ❐ Boat systems status

4

Keeping Watch

Rules of the Road/ Buoys

Vessel Lights

Sound & Distress Signals

KEEPING WATCH

STAY ON BOARD	STAY AFLOAT	STAY OUT OF THE WAY	STAY THE COURSE
❐ Use an attached harness when alone on watch and always keep it on when on deck.	❐ Inspect bilge and be attentive to bilge pump cycling.	❐ Keep a good lookout.	❐ Keep on course.
❐ If alone, ask next watch for help with sail changes or maneuvers.	❐ Inspect engine room.	❐ Use radar and AIS to determine risk of collision.	❐ Monitor chart for obstacles and markers on the course.
		❐ Alert skipper early about potential risk.	❐ Maintain speed and direction.
			❐ Listen to radio traffic and warnings.
			❐ Be alert to engine sensors, e.g., temperature, oil, and battery charging and status.
			❐ Log any departure from plan or routine.

WARNING!

- When in doubt or if action is required, alert skipper.
- Do not nap, sleep, or stay below longer than necessary for the ship business. If you cannot stay alert, wake up the following watch.

RULES OF THE ROAD/BUOYS

UNDER POWER

❒ Give way to:

- Sailing vessels
- Vessels engaged in fishing
- Vessels not under command
- Vessels limited by their ability to maneuver
- Vessels in traffic lane

❒ Meeting vessels under power:

HEAD ON

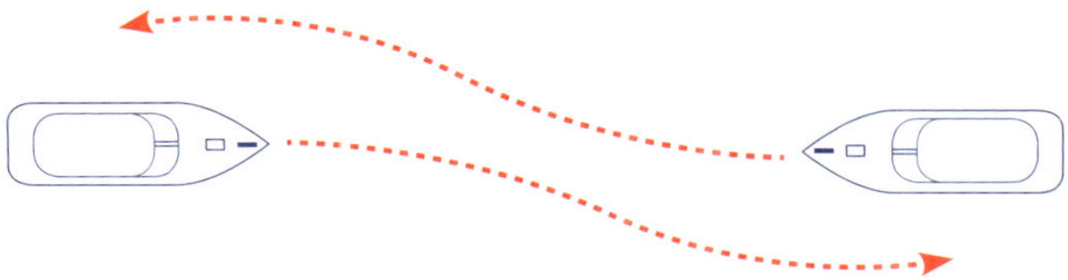

OVERTAKING

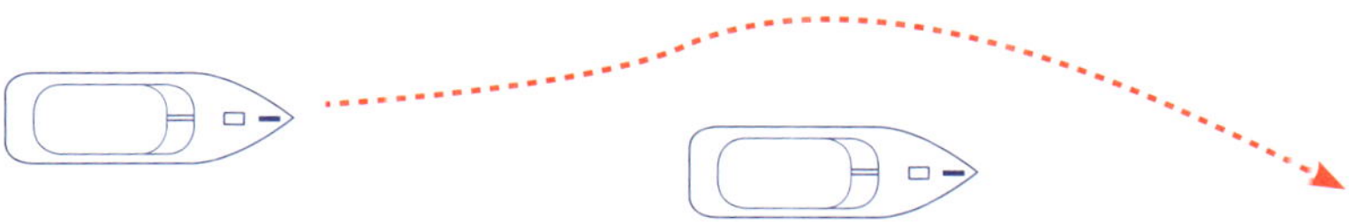

CROSSING

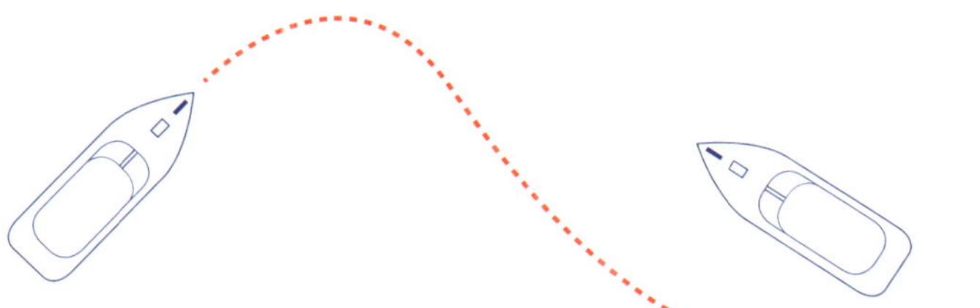

Continued On Next Page

NAVIGATIONAL BUOYS

LATERAL BUOYS AND MARKS

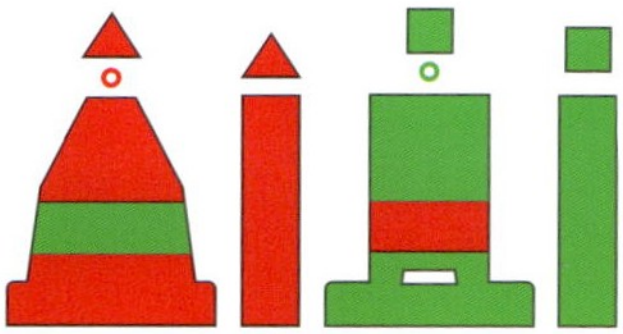

Define channel borders; indicate direction. These examples show IALA Region B, including the Americas. In Region A, the Green and Red change sides (e.g. Green, Right, Returning).

Moving Shoreward:

- Red, Right, Returning
- Red buoys to starboard side, even numbers; red nun or pillar shape
- Green buoys to port side, odd numbers; green can or pillar shape
- Numbers increase toward shore

Moving Seaward:

- Red buoy to port side, even numbers; nun or pillar shape
- Green buoys to starboard side, odd numbers; green can or pillar shape

PREFERRED CHANNEL MARKERS

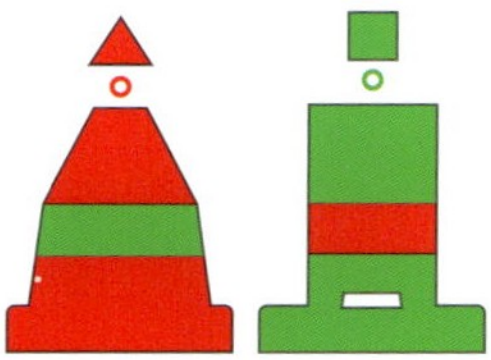

Horizontal bands of red and green; top color indicates the direction of the preferred channel.

- Top red (nun or pillar shape): keep marker to starboard if returning from sea
- Top green (can or pillar shape): keep marker to port if returning from sea

ISOLATED DANGER

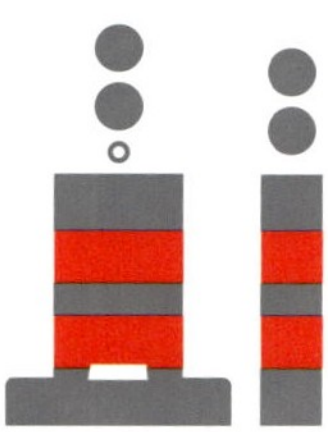

Body: Black with horizontal red bands
Top: 2 black spheres
Light (if present)**:** White flash

Continued On Next Page

SAFE WATER

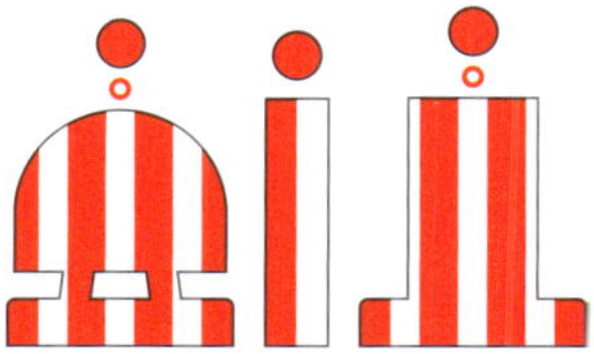

Body: Red and white vertical stripes
Top (if present)**:** 1 red sphere
Light (if present)**:** Calm and white

EMERGENCY WRECK

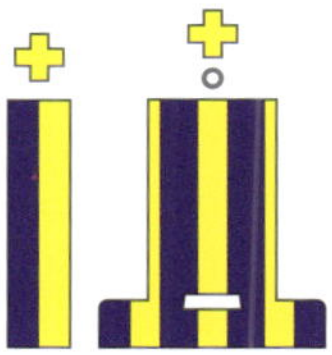

Body: Blue and yellow vertical stripes
Top (if present)**:** 1 yellow cross
Light (if present)**:** Alternating blue and yellow flash

CARDINAL BUOYS

Cardinal buoys show the position of a hazard and the direction of safe water. If lit, rhythms are either flashing Q (50 or 60 flashes per minute), or fast flashing VQ (100 or 120 flashes per minute).

WEST

The safest water lies to the west.
Markings: Yellow with central black band.
Top marks: Two stacked black cones, top one pointing down and bottom pointing up.
Light: White. VQ(9) followed by 10-second blackout, or Q(9) followed by 15-second blackout.

NORTH

The safest water lies to the north.
Markings: Top half black, bottom half yellow.
Top marks: Two stacked black cones, both pointing up.
Light: White. VQ or Q, continuous.

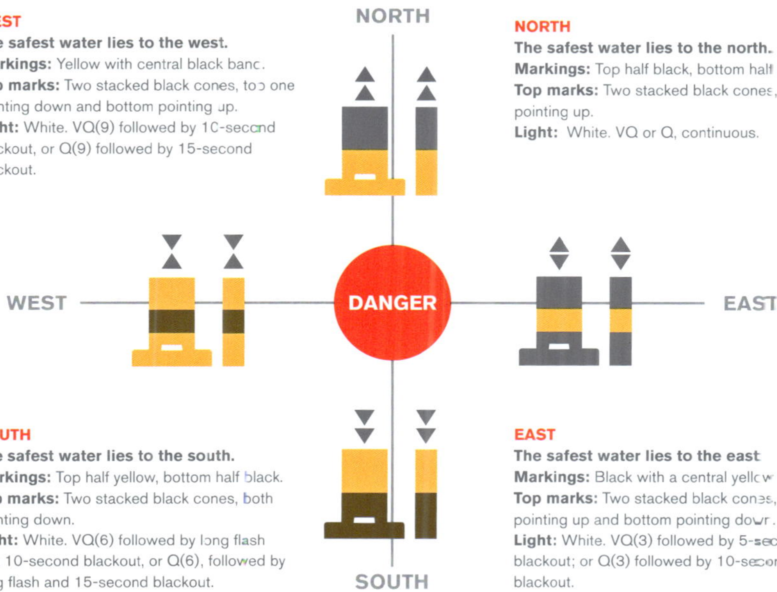

SOUTH

The safest water lies to the south.
Markings: Top half yellow, bottom half black.
Top marks: Two stacked black cones, both pointing down.
Light: White. VQ(6) followed by long flash and 10-second blackout, or Q(6), followed by long flash and 15-second blackout.

EAST

The safest water lies to the east
Markings: Black with a central yellow band.
Top marks: Two stacked black cones, top pointing up and bottom pointing down.
Light: White. VQ(3) followed by 5-second blackout; or Q(3) followed by 10-second blackout.

VESSEL LIGHTS

MOTOR VESSELS

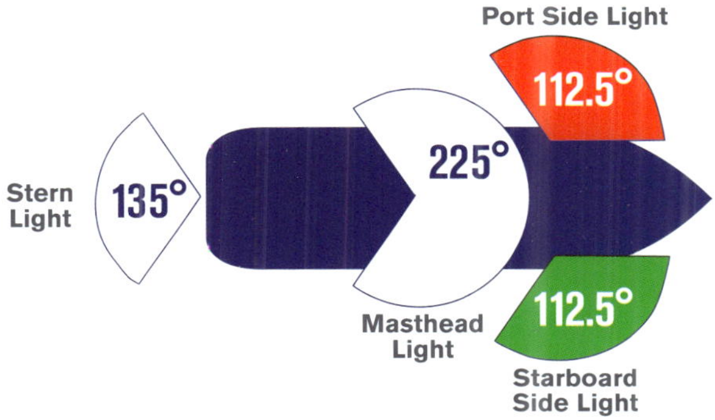

In addition, a vessel over 50m will show a second masthead light abaft and higher than the forward one.

SAILBOAT

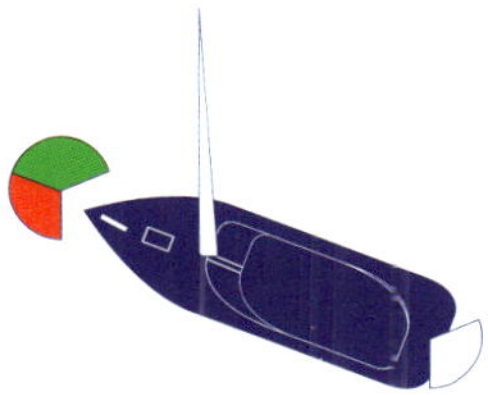

SAILBOAT UNDER POWER

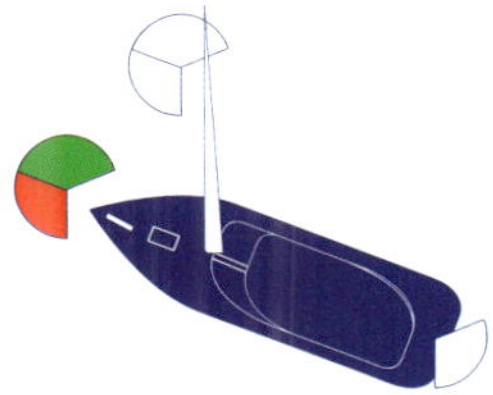

VESSEL ENGAGED IN FISHING

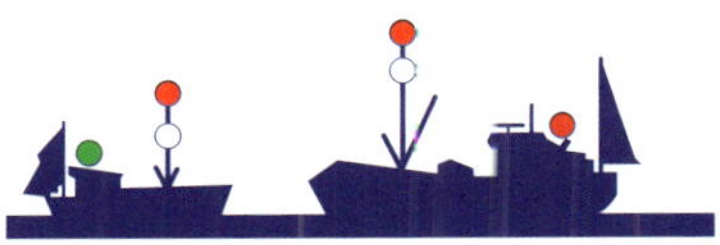

VESSEL TRAWLING

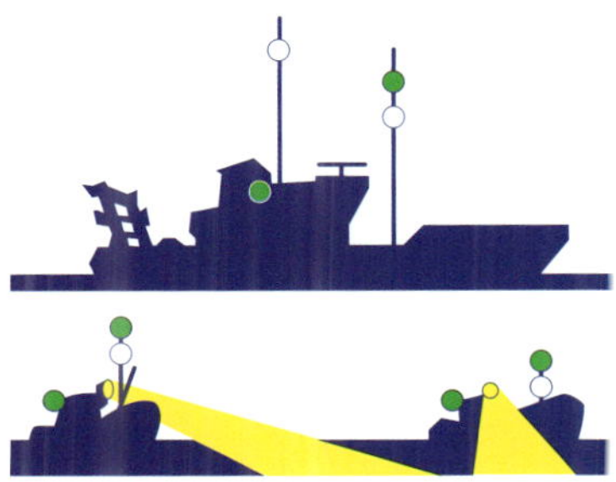

Continued On Next Page

VESSEL AT ANCHOR

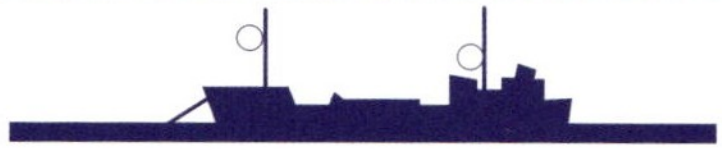

50m or more LOA:
Two all-round white lights

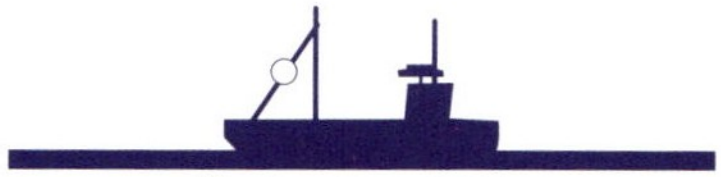

Under 50m LOA:
One all-round white light where best seen

VESSEL ON PILOTAGE DUTY

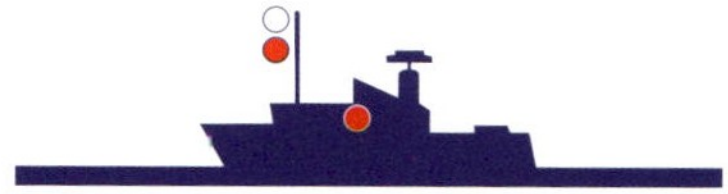

VESSEL CONSTRAINED BY DRAFT

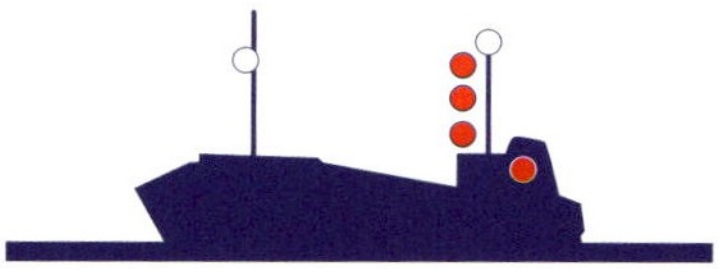

VESSEL NOT UNDER COMMAND

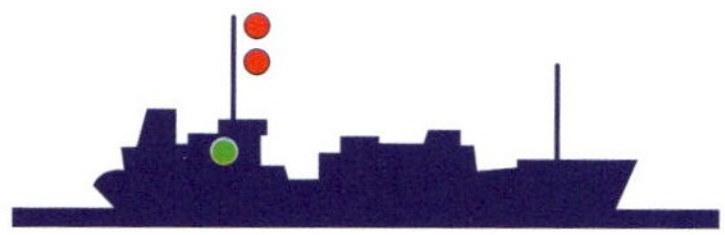

VESSEL AGROUND

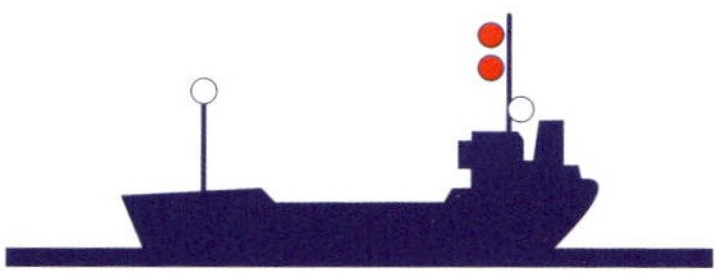

VESSEL TOWING

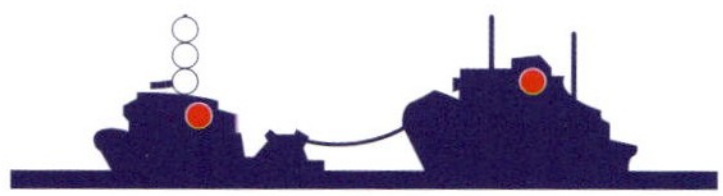

Bow Aspect

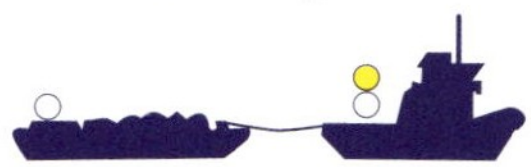

Stern Aspect

HOVERCRAFT

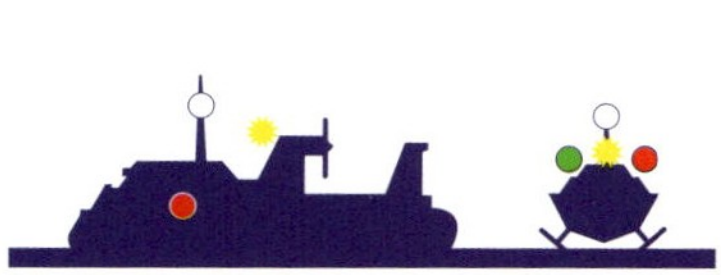

MINESWEEPING VESSEL

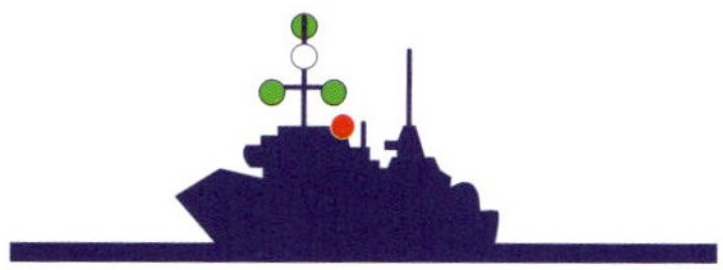

SOUND & DISTRESS SIGNALS

HORN OR WHISTLE

Short blast ● **(1 second)** Long blast ▬ **(4–6 seconds)**

VESSELS IN SIGHT OF EACH OTHER

- Turning to starboard ●
- Turning to port ● ●
- Engines in reverse ● ● ●
- Danger, I don't understand your intention ● ● ● ● ● (or more)

VESSELS IN NARROW CHANNEL

- Nearing blind turn ▬

  Intent to overtake:
  - To starboard ▬ ▬ ●
  - To port ▬ ▬ ● ●
- Agreement by other vessels ▬ ● ▬ ●

POOR VISIBILITY

Sounded at 2-minute intervals:

- Power vessels making way ▬
- Under way but not making way ▬ ▬

- Not under command (NUC)
- Restricted ability to maneuver (RAM)
- Constrained by draft (CBD)
- Vessel fishing
- Vessel towing or pushing

▬ ● ●

- Sailing vessel not using power
- Vessel under tow if manned

▬ ● ● ●

INTERNATIONAL DISTRESS SIGNALS

The spoken word "MAYDAY" sent by radiotelephony 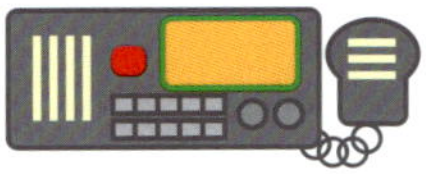	Rockets or shells throwing red stars at short intervals 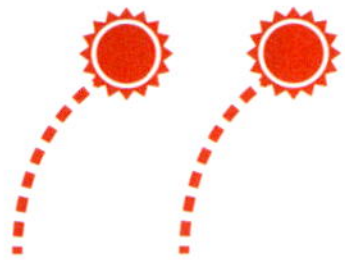
Wave outstretched arms slowly up and down 	Code Flags "N" and "C" 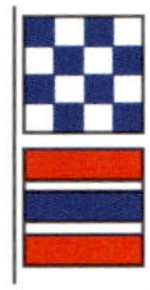
Red Parachute or Hand Flare 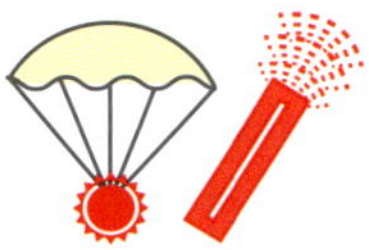	A Square Shape above or below a Ball Shape 
Orange Smoke 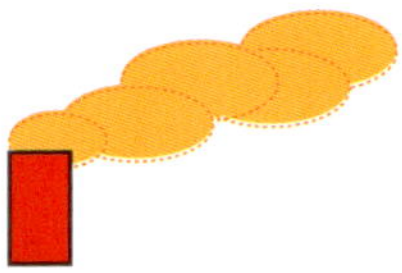	EPIRB Emergency Position Indicating Radio Beacon 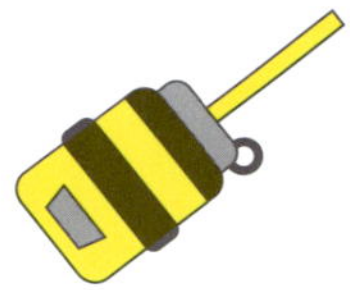
Morse S O S by radio or any other signalling method 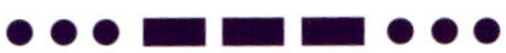	SART Radar Transponder 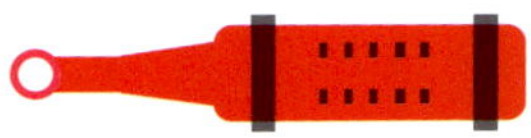
Gun or noise at 1 minute intervals 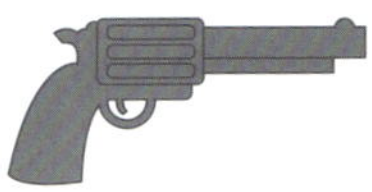	Radiotelegraph Alarm signal/ DSC 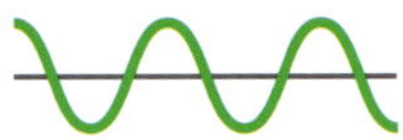
Continuous sound with fog signal 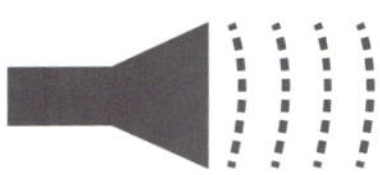	Radiotelephone Alarm Signal/ DSC 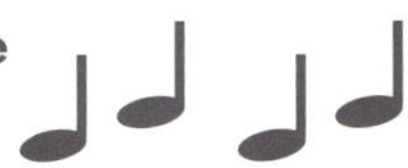
Flames or Smoke 	Dye Marker 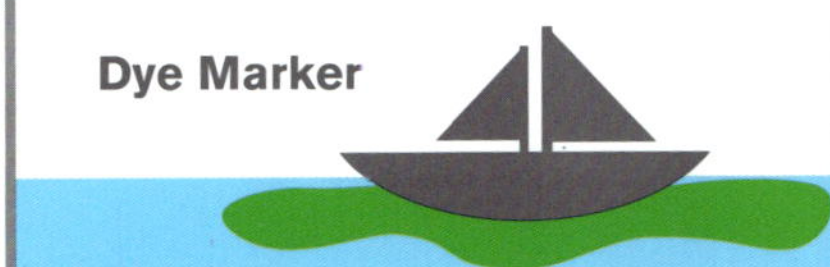

5. Heavy Weather Preparation

Systematic preparation for heavy weather goes a long way to focus energy, alleviate anxiety, and prepare the boat and crew.

FORECAST

- ❒ Consult several weather sources.
- ❒ Get local forecast and update frequently.
- ❒ Correlate the forecast with your observations of wind, barometer, clouds, and sea state.

CREW

- ❒ Prepare foul weather gear.
- ❒ Rig lee cloths on berths.
- ❒ Give everyone a good meal.
- ❒ Prepare sandwiches and a hot thermos.
- ❒ Issue seasickness pills.
- ❒ Brief crew on:
    - Safety on deck and in cockpit.
    - Sail reefing procedure.
    - Radio procedures.
    - Critical Equipment and Fittings.

    See 3. Critical Immediate-Access Equipment, p. 7; and See 9. Stow Plan, p. 29. ***(Safety Checklist)***

5

Continued On Next Page

ON DECK

- ❐ Remove dodger, spray hood, bimini, and flags.
- ❐ Consider rigging a rope lattice in cockpit.
- ❐ Put ready bag in cockpit with additional lines, blocks, flashlight, and multi-tool knife.
- ❐ Prepare drag devices, such as sea anchor or wraps.
- ❐ Stow inflatable dinghy.
- ❐ Put washboards, windowboards into position.
- ❐ Secure all gear on deck:
  - Anchors
  - Life raft
  - MOB gear

BELOW DECK

- ❐ Charge batteries.
- ❐ Consider changing gas cylinders and batteries of portable devices.
- ❐ Have engine filters ready.
- ❐ Top fuel.
- ❐ Secure all gear below deck:
  - Stove gimbals
  - Lockers
  - Drawers
  - Floorboards
  - Chart table
  - Wash boards
- ❐ Close all seacocks other than engine and bilge pump.
- ❐ Pump bilge.
- ❐ Check steering system.
- ❐ Check for manual bilge pump handles and secure to pumps.

6. Boat Specifications & Limitations

SPECIFICATIONS

Length OA (overall)	______________	
Length WL (waterline)	______________	
Beam	______________	
Draft	______________	
Displacement	______________	
Height over water	______________	

LIMITATIONS

Cruising RPM	______________	
Cruising speed	______________	
Max speed RPM	______________	
Hull speed	______________	
Water tank(s)	______________	
Fuel tank(s)	______________	
Miles per liter	______________	1/sm
Max range on full fuel tank	______________	
Engine service hours interval	______________	h

7. Engine Diagram

Insert details of your boat's engine.

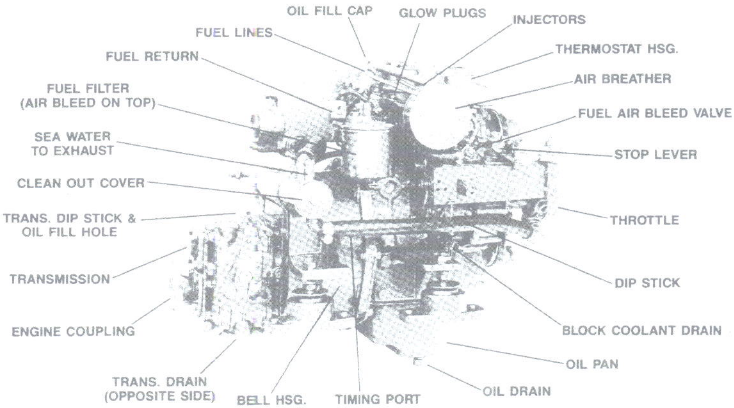

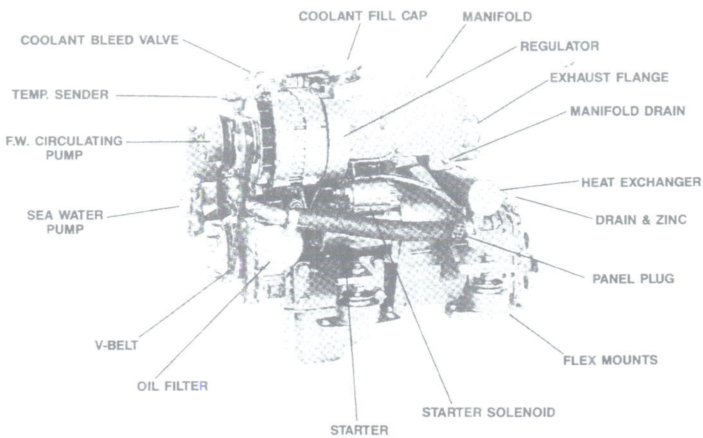

8. Deck Plan

Insert sketches of your own boat's deck plan.

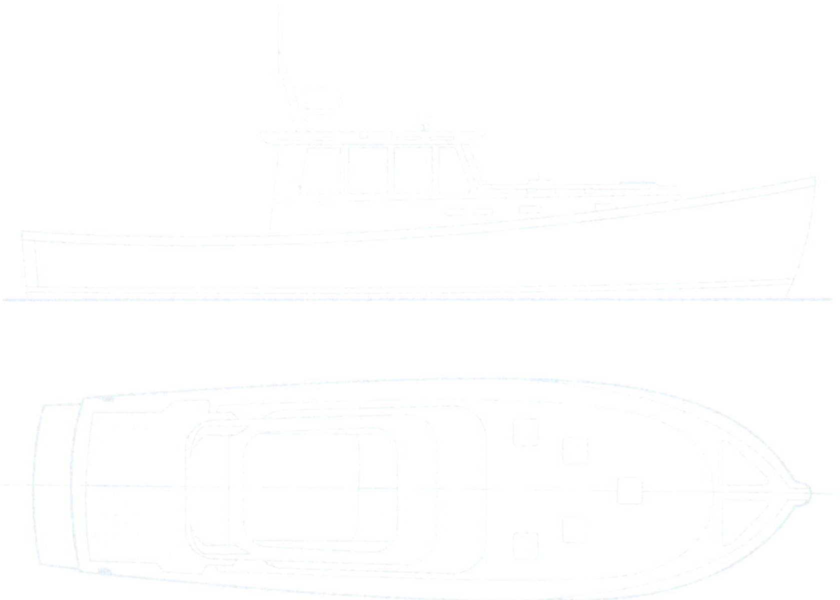

8

9. Stow Plan for Critical Equipment & Fittings

Insert sketches of your own ship's stow plan.

See 3. Critical Immediate-Access Equipment, p. 7 ***(Safety Checklist)***

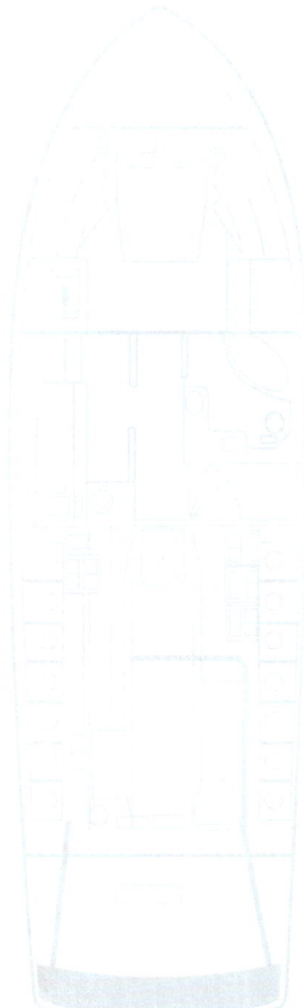

9

10. Fuel Consumption

Insert the appropriate values for your engine(s)

Total fuel capacity: ________________ **Usable capacity:** ________________

Safety margin (in percentage): ________ **Fuel price per gallon:** ________________

Speed in knots in calm water	Consumption: Gallons/hour	Consumption: Miles/gallon	Motoring range	Consumption in $/hour	Consumption in $/mile	RPM
4						
6						
8						
10						
12						
14						
16						
18						
20						
22						
24						

11. Kits

Damage Control

Medical

Boat Tools & Spares

Engine Mainte-nance

Kits

DAMAGE CONTROL

DEDICATED DAMAGE CONTROL KIT

- ❒ Soft wood plugs stowed next to all through-hulls
- ❒ Underwater-curing epoxy
- ❒ Wooden wedges and blocks of various sizes
- ❒ Packing and wrenches for shaft log
- ❒ Caulking materials
- ❒ Collision mat
- ❒ Plastic sheets
- ❒ Pumps and bailing containers

AD HOC KIT

Parts and materials that have other uses on the boat but can be used in an emergency for damage control:

- ❒ Floor boards of various sizes
- ❒ Cabin doors
- ❒ Mattresses
- ❒ Boat poles
- ❒ Plastic bags
- ❒ Duct tape
- ❒ Soft steel wire and Dacron twine
- ❒ Fasteners
- ❒ Fiberglass and epoxy components
- ❒ Hose clamps of all size, hoses, inner tube rubber

MEDICAL KIT

MEDICAL EQUIPMENT

- ❒ 12 Nitrile examination gloves
- ❒ 3 Antimicrobial hand wipes
- ❒ 1 Blood pressure cuff
- ❒ 1 Stethoscope
- ❒ 1 Oral airway kit (set of 6)
- ❒ 2 Surgical gloves 7.5mm
- ❒ 1 Digital thermometer 90°–105°F
- ❒ 1 Clothing shears
- ❒ 1 Splinter picker forceps
- ❒ 6 Safety pins
- ❒ 1 Emergency reflective blanket

MEDICAL SUPPLIES

- ❒ 4 Antimicrobial hand wipes
- ❒ 1 Surgical scrub brush
- ❒ 2 Povidone iodine solution (1 oz.)
- ❒ 20 Wound closure strips (butterfly strips)
- ❒ 4 Tincture of benzoin
- ❒ 1 Antibiotic ointment 1oz.
- ❒ 8 Antibiotic ointment packets
- ❒ 20 After Cuts & Scrapes® wipes
- ❒ 15 Alcohol swabs
- ❒ 72 4×4 or 3×3 or 2×2s sterile dressings
- ❒ 10 4x4 non-sterile dressings
- ❒ 10 Antimicrobial hand wipes
- ❒ 1 Self-Adherent elastic bandage 2" (Coban or other)
- ❒ 2 Eye pads
- ❒ 5 Non-adherent sterile dressings
- ❒ 2 Adaptic® non-adherant dressings

Continued On Next Page

- ❒ 3 Conforming gauze bandages (2" or 3")
- ❒ 2 Adhesive tape: 10 yards (1")
- ❒ 42 Strip, knuckle & fingertip bandages
- ❒ 8 Waterproof bandages
- ❒ 40 Cotton-tipped applicators
- ❒ 1 Moleskin 7" × 4"
- ❒ 4 Tongue blades
- ❒ 1 Scalpel #11, blade sterile
- ❒ 2 Self-adherent elastic bandages 3" & 2"

BURN TREATMENT

- ❒ 2 Nitrile gloves
- ❒ 2 Aloe gel
- ❒ 1 Spenco 2nd® Skin 2" × 3"
- ❒ 1 Spenco 2nd® Skin 3" × 4"
- ❒ 4 Adaptic® non-adherent dressings
- ❒ 2 Non-woven adhesive knit bandages
- ❒ 1 Self-adherent elastic nandage

EXTREMITY TRAUMA

- ❒ 1 SAM® splint
- ❒ 2 SAM® finger splint
- ❒ 2 Instant cold compresses
- ❒ 2 Elastic bandages with Velcro® (4" or 6")
- ❒ 1 Self-adherent elastic bandage 3"
- ❒ 2 Triangular bandages
- ❒ 1 Neck collar for immobilization
- ❒ 1 Inflatable arm splint
- ❒ 1 Inflatable leg splint

Continued On Next Page

OVER-THE-COUNTER MEDICATION

- ❒ 3 Oral rehydration mix packages
- ❒ 1 Ear drops
- ❒ 2 Eye wash
- ❒ 6 Medique® Alamag Plus antacid
- ❒ 24 Acetaminophen (325 mg)
- ❒ 50 Ibuprofen (200 mg)
- ❒ 12 Aspirin (325mg)
- ❒ 12 Antihistamine
- ❒ 12 Imodium AD®
- ❒ 6 Cortisone cream 1%
- ❒ 6 Pepcid® AC
- ❒ 20 Meclizine (Antivert, 25 mg)
- ❒ 20 Diphenhydramine 25 mg
- ❒ 20 Chlorpheneramine
- ❒ 1 Antibacterial Hand Gel

PRESCRIPTION MEDICATION

- ❒ 30 Norco 5/325 for severe pain relief
- ❒ 28 Trimethoprim Sulfamethoxazole (Bactrim DS) antibiotic
- ❒ 40 Amoxicillin Clavulinic Acid (Augmentin 250) antibiotic
- ❒ 28 Ciprofloxacin (500 mg) antibiotic
- ❒ 3 Azithromycin 6 pak (Z-pak) antibiotic
- ❒ 1 60 gram Silvadene antibiotic burn ointment

BOAT TOOLS

- ❒ Allen wrenches for all sizes of Allen screws on board
- ❒ Chisels, cold and wood
- ❒ Hand drill with bits set
- ❒ Electric drill with bits set
- ❒ Metal files set
- ❒ Wood files set
- ❒ Hammers: 5 pound; 2 pound; ballpeen; clew
- ❒ Mallet
- ❒ Pliers set, flat and needle-nose in assorted sizes
- ❒ Putty knives
- ❒ Saws: Metal; wood; jigsaw; spare blades
- ❒ Screw drivers: Flat and Phillips; assorted sizes
- ❒ Tin snips
- ❒ Vise
- ❒ Wire brushes

BOAT SPARES

- ❒ Water pump
- ❒ Bilge pump
- ❒ Had servicing kit
- ❒ Repair kits for pumps

- ❒ Electrical wire, assorted size and length
- ❒ Soft iron sizing wire
- ❒ Assorted hoses
- ❒ Assorted hose clamps
- ❒ Duct tape
- ❒ 2-part epoxy
- ❒ Silicone sealant

Continued On Next Page

- ❒ Silicone lubricant spray and grease
- ❒ O-ring set

- ❒ Nuts, bolts, washers
- ❒ Sandpaper, wet and dry
- ❒ Pacing for shaft and rubber glands

- ❒ Snap shackles
- ❒ D shackles
- ❒ Assorted blocks and connectors
- ❒ Spare anchor chain or line

ENGINE MAINTENANCE KIT

BASIC TOOLS

- ❒ Box and wrench set for all American and metric bolts on board
- ❒ Vice grips
- ❒ Pipe wrench
- ❒ Pliers set
- ❒ Phillips and slotted screwdriver sets
- ❒ Hacksaw and blades
- ❒ Punches and chisels
- ❒ Hammers, large and small
- ❒ Measuring tools: tape, ruler, feelers, caliper
- ❒ Metal files
- ❒ Strap wrench

SPARES

- ❒ Full set of fuel and oil filters for engines and generator
- ❒ Engine oil sufficient for a full oil change
- ❒ Oil filter wrench
- ❒ Raw water pump impeller
- ❒ Antifreeze, full change
- ❒ Transmit ion oil, full change
- ❒ Hydraulic oil, full refill
- ❒ 10 feet hydraulic hose and fitting
- ❒ Grease
- ❒ WD-40
- ❒ Gaskets material and liquid gasket
- ❒ Packing for stuffing box
- ❒ Spare set of engine belts
- ❒ Soldering kit

Continued On Next Page

ELECTRICAL

- ❒ Multimeter
- ❒ Test light
- ❒ Full set of connectors and a crimper
- ❒ Isolation tape
- ❒ Heat shrink tubes
- ❒ Electric ties
- ❒ Soldering kit
- ❒ Spare light bulbs for house and nav lights
- ❒ Fuses for all instruments
- ❒ Conductivity spray (more W-40)
- ❒ Flashlights, bulbs, and batteries

12. Equipment Lists & Contacts

12

SEAWISE

SeaWise is a creative enterprise dedicated to making action guide books and applications for the marine industry. The action guide series is a product of extensive research and experience as well as the integration of aviation concepts into the world of yacht sailing. The founders are two friends with a passion for sailing and a unique combination of skills.

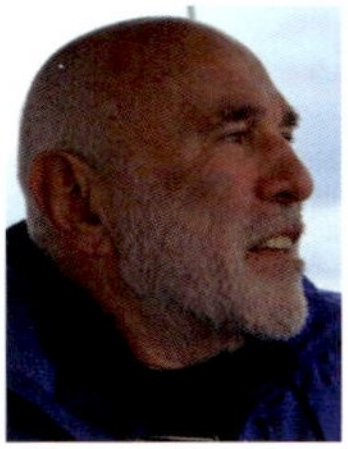

ZVI RICHARD DOR-NER

Zvi has sailed all his life on a variety of crafts and seas. When not sailing, he was a cameramen, director, and, for 30 years, an executive producer of documentary films for PBS, receiving multiple Emmy and other prestigious awards. Among others, he produced *Columbus and the Age of Discovery* and wrote the companion book. During the production, he sailed the replicas of Columbus's fleet in the Mediterranean and in the Atlantic. On his boat he crossed the Atlantic in both directions, sailed the Atlantic coasts of Europe and North America, and crisscrossed the Mediterranean and Caribbean. Zvi is qualified as a Yachtmaster Offshore by the RYA and holds a US Coast Guard Master 100 Ton License with Sail Endorsement. Much of this guide was written on his 43-foot ketch *S/V Nina*.

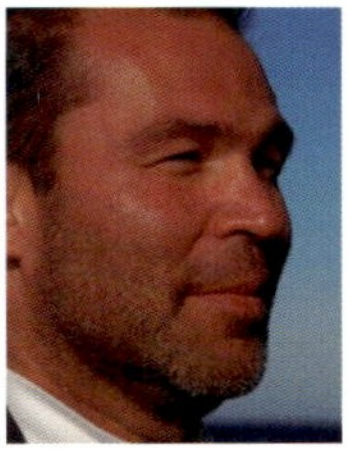

ZVI FRANK

When he doesn't sail, Frank is a high-tech and social media entrepreneur. He is the executive chairman of Zemingo Mobile Group, a company specializing in mobile applications design, development, and marketing. Previously, Frank founded and led a high-tech web conferencing company in the US that was later acquired by AT&T. Frank is also an active film producer and won an Emmy award for co-producing the documentary *Google Baby*. He has served as an officer and an F-16 fighter pilot and flight instructor in the Israeli Air Force. He is a qualified skipper and sails extensively with his family on his 54-foot sloop *S/Y Genesis*, where the remaining parts of this guide were written.

SeaWise

EMERGENCY ACTION GUIDE

FOR MOTOR YACHTS

Flooding

Collision

Running Aground

Fire

Loss of Steering

Engine Failure

Medical Emergency

Man Overboard

Extreme Weather

Abandon Ship

Rescue

Skipper Disabled

Emergency Communications

Foreword

Emergencies at sea require fast and appropriate action. The two-part SeaWise guide provides concise and direct guidance for preparing for and dealing with emergencies.

The Emergency Action part of the guide should be used by skippers before voyages to review and practice crew responses to emergency situations. Skippers can teach important standard procedures, while allowing for vessel-specific adaptations as needed. When situations arise at sea, the guide provides immediate, step-by-step instruction.

The Checklist provides a systematic way to prepare a well-founded boat for voyaging and enable a competent crew to deal effectively with emergencies.

SeaWise Action Guide is based on extensive research and a great deal of experience; yet, it is only a guide. The sea, in its infinite forms, as well as the variety of boats, equipment, and crews will make every emergency unique. It is the responsibility of skippers to integrate this guide with all they know, to apply their knowledge to the specific circumstance, and to command their ships to safety. It is a responsibility that the authors cannot share.

1. Flooding

Consider the volume of water coming in and your ability to pump water out. Focus first on stopping the flooding, then on removing the water.

1

INDICATORS

- Water inside the boat
- Bilge alarm sounding
- Bilge pumps cycling

IMMEDIATE ACTIONS

Taste the water in the boat.

- **If fresh water: no emergency.**

- **If salt water:**
  - **Relieve pressure on the boat** by slowing down to steering speed.
  - **Turn on bilge pump** and activate any emergency pumps.
  - **Start engine** and keep it in neutral.
  - **Consider changing course** and heading toward help or beaching.
  - **Establish benchmark** for the water level.

Continued On Next Page

CHECK & ACT

1 Check if cooling water is **pulsating** normally from the exhaust port.

If cooling water IS NOT pulsating:

Suspect the engine salt-water system, and check:

- **a)** Engine seacock
- **b)** Raw water filter
- **c)** Raw water impeller
- **d)** Raw water hoses
- **e)** Exhaust hoses
- **f)** Exhaust muffler

▶ Identify the leak.

Try to repair without shutting down the engine If the leak is below pumps, wait.

If cooling water IS pulsating:

Close all seacocks **except** the engine raw/salt-water seacock.

2 If flooding stops:

- **a)** Check if any toilet bowls are full; suspect the system.
- **b)** Identify the damaged system by opening and closing each of the seacocks individually.

▶ Repair as needed

3 If flooding persists:

Inspect all remaining through-hull fittings.

- **a)** Bilge pump hoses
- **b)** Stuffing box
- **c)** Rudder shaft
- **d)** Tank fills and vents
- **e)** Transducers and sensors
- **f)** Bow thruster
- **g)** Generator raw water and exhaust
- **h)** Air-conditioning cooling water system

▶ Repair as needed

Continued On Next Page

Note: In extreme weather, also check on-deck fittings: hull-to-deck joints, hatches, cockpit drains, hawse pipe, and anchor locker.

Note: Unless you were involved in a collision or sustained structural damage, continue systematically checking the systems connected to the sea; it will pay off.

4 If flooding continues:

a) Transmit a **Pan-Pan.**

See 7. Emergency Communications, p. 37. ***(Action Guide)***

b) Maximize water-expelling efforts by managing crew resources to:

- Use manual pumps
- Bail
- Close engine seacock and redirect engine raw water intake to pump from inside the boat
- Use external pumps if available from other vessels

5 If water continues to rise:

a) Transmit **Mayday**

See 7. Emergency Communications, p. 37. ***(Action Guide)***

b) Prepare to **Abandon Ship**

See 11. Abandon Ship, p. 83. ***(Action Guide)***

Flooding

Flooding

2. Collision

In a collision, identifying the point of impact and locating a possible hull breach provide the most important information about what needs to be done.

Be prepared with a crowbar to remove paneling and furniture to access the damaged area.

Distinguish between collision and grounding.

See 3. Running Aground, p. 11. ***(Action Guide)***

2

INDICATORS

- Impact
- Sound
- Deceleration
- Change of direction
- Crew report

IMMEDIATE ACTIONS

- **Check** that all crew is safe on board.
  See 9. Man Overboard, p. 67. ***(Action Guide)***
- **Check** if anyone sustained injuries — if so, deal with it.
  See 8. Medical Emergency, p. 47. ***(Action Guide)***
- **Identify** point of impact.
- **Check bilge.**
- **Assess** damage.
- **Initiate radio** contact if Mayday condition is developing

Continued On Next Page

- **If water is coming in:**
  - **Maneuver** to keep the breach above waterline if possible.
  - **Isolate the breach** by locking water-tight doors and passages.
  - **Turn on bilge pump** and activate any emergency pumps.
  - **Consider changing course** toward help or soft beaching.
  - **Establish benchmarks** for the water level.

CHECK & ACT

1 **Analyze breach** size and form, clear area for work, and consider working from outside.

- **If the breach is small:**

  See 11. Kits, p. 33. ***(Safety Checklist)***

  - Stuff materials such as softwood tapered plugs, patches, gasket material, and a closed foam pillow against the breach or inflate a life jacket inside the breach. Back the patch with plywood. Use wedges and poles to press the plywood against the breach. Apply plastic sheets and caulking to increase water tightness

- **If the breach is large:**
  - Prepare a plug on deck and consider patching it on top of the breach from outside of the boat. Take a floorboard, a door or a hatch cover larger than the hole, cover it with a closed-cell foam mattress or pillow, and pierce the two in the middle. With a line, make a thick stop knot and run it through a hole in the floorboard and closed-cell foam. Prepare a swimmer to pass the end of the line through the breach. Tighten the floorboard with the foam toward the hull, on the hole, and secure the line inside the boat. Use caulking with underwater epoxy to make it watertight.

Continued On Next Page

If the breach is irregular and larger than what a floorboard will cover:

- Lower a collision mat, a plastic sheet or a sail, preferably from the bow aft, while securing all end points with lines. Adjust the sheet to cover the breach and tie all lines and then continue to secure the breach from inside.

2 **If flooding continues:**

Maximize water-expelling and manage crew to:

a) Use manual pumps.

b) Bail.

c) Use external pumps from other vessels.

d) Close engine seacock and redirect engine raw water intake to pump from inside the boat.

Note: Do not stop fighting the breach and repairing the leak. Do **not** abandon ship until it is sinking.

3 **When flooding stops or you are in control of the flood, cancel any emergency communications transmitted.**

4 **If the water keeps rising:**

a) Transmit **Mayday.**

See 7. Emergency Communications, p. 37. ***(Action Guide)***

b) Prepare to **Abandon Ship.**

See 11. Abandon Ship, p. 83. ***(Action Guide)***

c) If close to shore, consider beaching the boat.

3. Running Aground

In shallow water, navigate at low speed and be constantly aware of the depth of the water and the effect of tides and current. Do not rely on a single source of information.

Soft grounding in sheltered waters is not dangerous. But grounding on a lee shore in heavy weather can lead to a total loss

INDICATORS

- Boat hits the ground
- Motion suddenly stops
- Taking on water
- Loss of steering

3

IMMEDIATE ACTIONS

On first touch, stop. Then if power train is free of the bottom, use all power in reverse.

When hard aground:

1 Put the engine in neutral.
2 Inspect bilge for incoming water.
3 If near an active waterway, transmit **Sécurité** message **on being aground.**

See 7. Emergency Communications, p. 37. ***(Action Guide)***

Continued On Next Page

CHECK & ACT

- **If the boat is taking on water:**
  Keep the boat aground until you repair the leak.
  Consider repairing from the outside.
  See 2. Collision, p. 7. ***(Action Guide)***

- **If the boat is not taking on water:**
  Determine, by direct observation and tide tables, if the tide is ebbing or flooding.

- **If tide is significant and is flooding:**
  Drop anchor up tide and wait to be lifted off ground.

- **If tide is significant and is ebbing:**
  Consider waiting until next flood and prepare for even lower water:
  a) Attempt to lean the boat toward higher ground.
  b) Deploy anchor(s) in the direction of deep water and protect the hull as it touches bottom. Place fenders, floorboards, cushions, and mattresses between the hull and ground.
  c) Attempt to protect the shaft(s), strut(s), propeller(s) and the rudder(s).
  d) When the tide floods, secure hatches and companionway from the rising water until the hull floats.

- **If tide is insignificant:**
  a) Survey for deep water and plan the direction of extraction.
  b) Place an anchor in the direction of extraction.
  c) Make sure the running gear is free of the bottom.
  d) Apply full tension to the anchors and back up on the engine to apply power and to create a prop-wash to free the hull.

Continued On Next Page

If the running gear (either prop, shaft, or struts) is locked or damaged, you need outside help.

- **If another boat is available, ask the skipper to:**
  a) Tow you into deep water.
  b) Carry your anchor into deeper water.
  c) Create a wake for "touch-and-go" movement.

- **If unable to extract:**
  Transmit a **Pan-Pan** and ask for help.
  See 7. Emergency Communications, p. 37. ***(Action Guide)***

- **When extracted:**

1 Inspect bilge for incoming water.
2 Inspect running gear and rudder operation.
3 Make sure engine cooling water intake is open.

4. Fire

Fire is sustained by fuel, oxygen, and heat. When fighting a fire, try to eliminate or diminish as much of these as possible.

Treat even a small fire as a major emergency. Fire spreads fast and can easily get out of control

Have some fire extinguishers accessible from the cockpit.

Consider a firm policy of no smoking on board and no unattended flames.

INDICATORS

- Flames or smoke
- Smell of smoldering electric insulation
- Fire alarm
- Temperature increase

Fire in Engine ↓

Fire in Galley ↓

Fire in Cabin/ on Deck ↓

FIRE IN ENGINE

IMMEDIATE ACTIONS

- **Check** that no crew is trapped by fire.
- **Stop engine** (if not done automatically).
- **Shut off** engine fuel and cooking gas.

CHECK & ACT

1 Activate any automatic fire extinguishing system.
See 9. Stow Plan, p. 29. ***(Safety Checklist)***

2 Keep adequate electricity to operate communication equipment; cut off everything else.

2 Keep the engine room closed to minimize oxygen inflow.

3 Insert fire extinguisher's nozzle through access port directly into the engine room.

4 **Remove flammable material** that might feed the fire.

5 **Consider transmitting Mayday.**
See 7. Emergency Communications, p. 37. ***(Action Guide)***

WARNING!
Never use water on electrical or fuel fire!

6 **If fire persists and spreads:**

a) Transmit **Mayday.**
See 7. Emergency Communications, p. 37. ***(Action Guide)***

b) Prepare to **Abandon Ship.**
See 11. Abandon Ship, p. 83. ***(Action Guide)***

FIRE IN GALLEY

IMMEDIATE ACTIONS

- **Check** that no crew is trapped by fire.
- **Slow engine** to steering speed only.
- **Shut off** cooking gas.
- **Keep adequate** electricity for radio operation, cut everything else.

CHECK & ACT

1 Activate any automatic galley fire extinguishing system.
See 9. Stow Plan, p. 29. ***(Safety Checklist)***

2 Attempt to smother the fire using:
- Wet towel
- Fire blanket
- Fire extinguisher

3 **Remove flammable material** that might feed the fire.

4 **Consider** transmitting **Mayday.**
See 7. Emergency Communications, p. 37. ***(Action Guide)***

WARNING!
Do not use water if fire is fueled by fat or oil!

5 **If fire persists and spreads:**

a) Transmit **Mayday**
See 7. Emergency Communications, p. 37. ***(Action Guide)***

b) Prepare to **Abandon Ship.**
See 11. Abandon Ship, p. 83. ***(Action Guide)***

FIRE IN CABIN / ON DECK

IMMEDIATE ACTIONS

- **Check** that no crew is trapped by fire.
- **Slow boat to steering speed only.**
- **Shut off** cooking gas.
- **Keep adequate** electricity for radio operation, cut everything else.

CHECK & ACT

1. **Maneuver** to keep the **fire downwind.**
2. **Escape** through forward or aft **hatches, shutting portholes and cabin doors** before (or after) exiting.
3. **Approach** the fire **from windward** aiming ABC fire extinguishers at the **base of the fire.**
4. **Use** water-hoses and buckets on any flammable material that produces ash.
5. **Remove flammable material** that might feed the fire.
6. Consider transmitting **Mayday.**

   See 7. Emergency Communications, p. 37. ***(Action Guide)***

7. **If fire persists and spreads:**

   a) Transmit **Mayday.**

   See 7. Emergency Communications, p. 37. ***(Action Guide)***

   b) Prepare to **Abandon Ship**

   See 11. Abandon Ship, p. 83. ***(Action Guide)***

5. Loss of Steering

During preparations for every departure, check the steering system before casting off mooring lines.
Turn the wheel hard over to starboard, and then hard over to port. Glance at the rudder. Note any interference and deal with it.

INDICATORS

- Steering wheel locked up
- Steering wheel not turning the rudder

5

In Close Quarters ↓

At Sea ↓

IN CLOSE QUARTERS

IMMEDIATE ACTIONS

1 Attempt to establish control by securing the boat to dock, buoy, or another boat using any means available.
   - Use engine to stop the boat.
   - Use bow thrusters for immediate maneuver.
   - Use combination of thruster and engine to trave.l
   - If twin engine, maneuver with engines.

   OR

2 Drop an anchor.

CHECK & ACT

- **If wheel is not turning:**
   - If autopilot is engaged, disengage it.
   - If quadrant is obstructed, clear it.

- **If wheel is not turning the rudder:**
   - Steer with bow thruster.
   - Steer with autopilot if it is connected directly to the quadrant.
   - Use emergency tiller

   See 3. Critical Equipment, p. 7. ***(Safety Checklist)***

- **If still unable to steer, consider:**
   - Using dinghy to push, tow, or direct the boat.
   - Hailing for help if within hailing distance.
   - Setting fenders and deck lines to protect from other boats and prepare for docking.
   - In traffic, transmit **Sécurité** "unable to maneuver" and ask for help.

   See 7. Emergency Communications, p. 37. ***(Action Guide)***

AT SEA

IMMEDIATE ACTIONS

1 Post a lookout.
2 **In traffic, transmit Sécurité** "out of control."
See 7. Emergency Communications, p. 37. ***(Action Guide)***
3 **Turn engine on.**

CHECK & ACT

- **If wheel is not turning:**
  - If autopilot is engaged, disengage it.
  - If wheel is locked, unlock it.
  - If quadrant is obstructed, clear it.

- **If wheel is not turning the rudder:**
  - Steer with autopilot if it is connected directly to the quadrant.
  - Use bow thruster and the engine for short-distance maneuvers.
  - Use emergency tiller.

See 3. Critical Equipment, p. 7. ***(Safety Checklist)***

- **If able to resume control:**
  - Set a safe course.
  - Examine and repair wheel-rudder connection, checking for cable system, hydraulic failure, or obstruction.

- **If rudder is jammed off center:**
  - Restore to center position by disconnecting mechanical or hydraulic damaged system.

OR

  - Wait for help or remove the rudder.

Continued On Next Page

- **If you have no working rudder, consider:**
  - Attaching a line directly to the drilled hole in the upper, outer part of the rudder, and move the rudder with these lines.
  - Build a makeshift rudder per your prepared plan and fittings.
  - Use the dinghy's outboard motor lashed directly to the stern or in combination with the dinghy for short distance maneuvering.
  - Revise your sailing plan to your situation.

- **If unable to achieve sufficient control,** transmit a **Pan Pan** and ask for help.

See 7. Emergency Communications, p. 37. ***(Action Guide)***

6. Engine Failure

Minimize engine failure by utmost attention to preventive maintenance and the quality of your fuel.

Make it a point to know your engine.

INDICATORS

- Engine stops working
- Engine cannot be started
- Engine must be turned off because of malfunction

In Close Quarters

At Sea

IN CLOSE QUARTERS

Focus on regaining control of the boat.

IMMEDIATE ACTIONS

- Secure the boat to another boat, a dock, or a buoy.
- Drop an anchor.
- Hail a passing boat for help.
- Use a dinghy to tow or push.
- Prepare lines and fenders for docking.
- In traffic, transmit Sécurité "out of control" and ask for help.

See 7. Emergency Communications, p. 37. ***(Action Guide)***

AT SEA

Focus your immediate efforts on regaining control by troubleshooting the engine.

IMMEDIATE ACTIONS

- **Post a lookout** to keep watch for help and warn of danger. .
- **Prepare to drop an anchor.**
- **Investigate** if the engine can be repaired at sea.
- **Transmit Pan-Pan to establish communications and seek advice.** *See 7. Emergency Communications, p. 37.* ***(Action Guide)***

CHECK & ACT

1 If the engine has been running and stopped:
Put the engine in neutral and attempt to restart.

▸ **If the engine starts, suspect obstruction to the propeller,** such as a line or fishing gear. You will need to dive to clear the obstruction.

▸ **If the propeller is unobstructed but the engine doesn't start or it starts and stops, suspect fuel delivery problem. Check:**

a) If primary fuel filter is clogged, change it.

b) If the fuel tank is empty, add fuel.

▸ **If the engine still doesn't start, suspect that air entered the fuel system,** and bleed the engine.

▸ **If the engine still doesn't start,** ensure air intake is not obstructed, by checking the air filter.

Continued On Next Page

2 If the engine doesn't start/crank after you stopped it at sea — suspect electrical problem.

a) Check that the engine kill switch is enabled.

b) Check that the engine is in neutral.

c) If you hear a solenoid click when trying to start, check the batteries. Charge if necessary, or switch to secondary battery bank, or engage emergency crossover of batteries.

d) Verify all contacts from the batteries, batteries' switch, starter, as well as the contacts from the engine switch to the starter are clean and tight. Tighten contacts and spray with contact spray (e.g. WD-40).

3 If the engine is overheating.

a) Reduce speed to steering speed and attempt to reach a safe place for repair.

b) Check if salt cooling water is **pulsating** normally from the exhaust port.

If the cooling water is pulsating:

- Wait for the engine to cool and add coolant if necessary.
- With adequate coolant, suspect a sticky thermostat and deal with it.

If the cooling water is not pulsating:

- Verify that engine raw water seacock is open and unobstructed.
- Verify that the raw water filter is not clogged.
- Verify that the raw water pump is functioning, check the impeller and the belt, and change if needed.
- Verify that raw water exhaust hoses are not obstructed.

Continued On Next Page

4 If unable to repair, you need professional help.

- **Transmit Pan-Pan or Mayday (depending on your predicament) and prepare for tow or rescue.** *See 7. Emergency Communications, p. 37.* ***(Action Guide)***
- Verify battery status and manage your electricity usage.
- If not generating electricity, ration electrical consumption but **maintain radio contact.**
- Plot your location on paper charts and prepare for DR navigation.
- Manage available food and water.

7. Emergency Communications

Before a voyage, identify the radio channels, frequencies, and telephone numbers of emergency contacts in the area in which you are sailing.

Secure an advocate (a trusted friend) ashore to represent you in case of emergency.

Train a crew member(s) to transmit in an emergency.

General

Mayday

Pan-Pan and Sécurité

GENERAL

EMERGENCY TRANSMISSIONS

MAYDAY: Distress Transmission
Used only when there is an immediate danger of loss of life and immediate assistance is needed.

PAN-PAN: Urgency Transmission
Used when there is a serious situation, a danger to life or vessel, but immediate assistance is not required, e.g., for medical advice.

SÉCURITÉ: Safety Transmission
Used by authorities to convey messages of navigational hazard. You might use it when you observe a hazard or when your vessel becomes one.

WARNING!
It is illegal to use Mayday, Pan-Pan, and Sécurité except in an emergency!

OPERATING PROCEDURES

- **Use radio terminology:** Acknowledge, Over, Received, Say Again, Spell, Can't Read You, Roger, Standby, Station Calling, This Is, Wait, Out.
- **Use phonetic alphabet:** Alpha, Bravo, Charley, Delta, Echo, Foxtrot, Golf, Hotel, India, Juliet, Kilo, Lima, Mike, November, Oscar, Papa, Quebec, Romeo, Sierra, Tango, Uniform, Victor, Whiskey, X-ray, Yankee, Zulu.
- **Use phonetic numbering system:** Wun, Too, Three, Fo-wer, Five, Six, Sev-en, Ait, Nin-er, Zero.

Continued On Next Page

Transmit your distress signal on all means available and repeat until contact is established:

- **In Mayday situation, activate your 406 MHz EPIRB** (range global):
  - It transmits an emergency signal through satellite to SAR centers, which coordinate rescue operations around the globe. EPIRB identifies you and your location and provides a homing signal.

- **On VHF/DSC** (range 50 miles):
  - Select the type of distress from the menu provided and press the Distress button. It automatically issues a distress alarm to all vessels and authorities on VHF channel 70. It includes the nature of your distress, your MMSI address, and your GPS location.
  - Ch 16 (range up 20 miles).
  - Continue transmitting emergency communication.

- **On SSB 2182 KHz** (range 200-500 miles):
  - Press the emergency frequency button. It automatically alerts vessels and shore authorities to your broadcast.
  - The USCG has discontinued watch keeping on 2182. It now monitors 4125, 6215, 8291, and 12290. Choose an appropriate frequency for range and time of the day.

- **On satellite phone** (range global):
  - Follow your satellite service provider instructions for emergency calls and use the specific telephone number of closest SAR center or your land-based advocate.

Continued On Next Page

- **On cell phone** (range of GSM):
  - You need to know the telephone number of an SAR Center responsible for your area.
  - You need a local emergency number such as 911 in US (they should know how to connect you to CG/SAR, but it is not always fast) and your land-based advocate contact.

Note: A direction finder cannot home in on a satellite phone or cell phone. Using these, you must provide accurate coordinates.

MAYDAY

Use Mayday when a person or the vessel faces a grave and imminent danger and requires immediate assistance. Make sure your VHF is on high power.

1 Activate EPIRB

2 Transmit MAYDAY:

a) **Mayday—Mayday—Mayday**
b) Give your vessel name and its call sign. Repeat three times.
c) Give your GPS position or bearing and distance from known landmark.
d) State the nature of the emergency.
e) Give the number of people on board and state the condition of anybody injured.
f) Describe the seaworthiness of the vessel.
g) Describe the vessel.
h) Give the radio channel or frequency you will be listening to and the schedule.
i) **Over.**

Listen before repeating several times. If nobody responds, go to SSB, cell phone, or satellite phone.

3 On receiving a Mayday transmission:

You have a legal obligation to acknowledge, confirm, and act.

a) **Confirm** the name of the vessel sending the distress signals. Repeat three times.
b) Give your radio call signal and your vessel name. Repeat three times.
c) Acknowledge: **Received Mayday.**

Continued On Next Page

d) Pause and listen for other vessels responding to the Mayday. Establish which vessel is in best position or better equipped to provide assistance.

- **If it is you, act: contact the distressed vessel and give it your position and estimated time of arrival.**
- **If there is another vessel in a better position to render assistance, confirm that you will stand by.**

4 Relaying a Mayday transmission:

If you are the only one responding, relay the Mayday message to alert other vessels and maritime authorities to the Mayday, as you assist.

a) **Mayday Relay, Mayday Relay, Mayday Relay.**
b) Give your radio call signal and vessel name.
c) **Mayday Relay from__________.**
d) Give the position of the distressed vessel.
e) Provide information about the nature of distress and the vessel requiring assistance.
f) Give your position, state your intention, course, and speed.
g) Give the radio channel or frequency you will be listening to and the schedule.
h) **Over.** Listen for response. If none is given, keep repeating entire sequence as needed.

PAN-PAN

Use **Pan-Pan** in these situations:

- An urgent message forewarning the possibility of a serious danger developing, e.g., being swept in the direction of a lee shore without power or taking on water.
- When medical advice is needed.
- To receive needed advice about navigation.

Follow the procedure as a **Mayday** transmission, except precede the transmission with **Pan-Pan** and the nature of the problem:

a) **Pan-Pan—Pan-Pan—Pan-Pan**

b) Give your radio call signal and your vessel name. Repeat three times.

c) State the nature of the urgency, e.g., **Medico, I require medical advice.**

d) Give the radio channel or frequency you will be listening to and the schedule.

e) **Over**. Listen for response. If none is given, keep repeating entire sequence as needed.

A medical call will be patched to the Coast Guard fleet surgeon or a SAR center, who will decide if the injured or sick crew needs to be extracted or transferred.

Continued On Next Page

SÉCURITÉ

Maritime authorities use **Sécurité** transmissions to convey dangers to navigation, e.g.:

- A change in weather.
- A change in buoyage.
- A drifting container.

You should use **Sécurité** in these situations:

- To warn about a danger to navigation, such as a drifting vessel.
- When **your vessel** is a danger to navigation, e.g., your boat is out of control, you are forced to anchor in a free way, or you do not have working navigation lights in traffic.

Follow the exact same procedure as a **Mayday** transmission, except precede the transmission with **Sécurité** and the nature of the problem, e.g.:

a) **Sécurité—Sécurité—Sécurité**

b) Give your radio call signal, your vessel name and position. Repeat three times.

c) State the nature of the urgency, e.g., **I see a drifting container, I am adrift.**

8. Medical Emergency

You should know the medical history, current state of health, and physical limitations of all people on board.

IMMEDIATE ACTIONS

- **Remove injured crew from danger**.
- **Sail the boat** on a safe course.
- **Administer first aid**.
- **Consider** changing course toward help.

- Drowning
- Head Injury
- Injury to Limb
- Confusion & Lethargy Hypothermia, Heat Stroke, Seasickness
- Burns
- Chest Pain/Heart Attack
- Injury to Trunk
- Allergic Reactions and Stings

DROWNING

INDICATORS

- Immersion in water
- Not breathing

IMMEDIATE ACTIONS

- **Stabilize victim** by placing on a hard flat surface.
- **Administer CPR**, but if you suspect hypothermia, once stable, remove wet clothing and cover with dry, warm blanket.

CHECK & ACT

1. Shake victim and shout "Can you hear me?"
2. If no response, **DO NOT DELAY, DO NOT CHECK FOR BREATHING OR PULSE,** begin CPR
3. Have a crew member establish **MAYDAY** contact and state that CPR is in progress

   See 7. Emergency Communications, p. 37. ***(Action Guide)***
4. ▸ **If you ARE NOT TRAINED in CPR**, begin chest compressions with hands placed in the middle of the chest at nipple line at the rate of 100/minute. Continue until help arrives.

   ▸ **If you ARE TRAINED in CPR,** begin chest compressions with hands placed in the middle of the chest at nipple line at the rate of 100/minute. Give 30 compressions. Then open the victim's airway using head tilt, chin lift procedure.
   - Give two breaths sufficient to cause the chest to rise.
   - Breaths are about 1 second each.
   - Be sure the chest rises with ventilations.

   Give 30 compressions, then two more ventilations, doing this approximately 3 cycles per minute for a total of about 2 minutes.

Continued On Next Page

5 If an automatic electronic defibrillator (AED) is available, use it at this time.
6 If you are alone, place **MAYDAY** call after first two minutes of CPR, and then return to CPR as quickly as possible.
See 7. Emergency Communications, p. 37. ***(Action Guide)***
7 Continue CPR as long as you and the crew can maintain the effort or until help arrives; recovery may be delayed especially in cold water drowning.

BURNS

Most burns on boats are due to sun, heat, or flame. The goals are to reduce pain, protect against infection, and provide medical attention, as needed.

INDICATORS

Burns are judged by two basic criteria: depth and extent.

a) The depth of the burn determines the damage to the skin
- 1st degree or superficial affects the outer layer of skin (sunburn).
- 2nd degree or partial thickness extends through the outer skin layer into the inner layer, and causes blistering or weeping (hot water scald).
- 3rd degree or full thickness extends through the skin layers to fat or muscle, and may appear waxy, pearly gray, or charred (clothing on fire).

b) Extent is expressed in percentage of body area, one palm of the victim equal to 1% of total body surface area)

Continued On Next Page

IMMEDIATE ACTIONS

- **Remove** the cause of the burn.
- **Cool the area** with clean water.
- **Give pain medication**, as needed (ibuprofen, acetaminophen, or narcotics).

CHECK & ACT

Determine the depth and percentage of burn to the total body surface area.

1 1st degree superficial burns can be managed with topical moisturizer, aloe vera gel, topical pain relievers, and ibuprofen or acetaminophen.

2 Limited 2nd degree partial thickness burns of <1% surface area:
   - May be treated as 1st degree burns.
   - DO NOT open the blister, as it protects from infection.
   - Use Silvadene cream and keep covered with sterile non-adhesive dressing changed daily.

3 More extensive 2nd degree burns of >1% but <20% surface area:
   - Treat as limited 2nd degree.

4 All 3rd degree full thickness burns and 2nd degree burns of >20% surface area:
   - Treat as limited 2nd degree.

5 Call **PAN-PAN** for medical advice and prepare for evacuation.
See 7. Emergency Communications, p. 37. ***(Action Guide)***

HEAD INJURY

INDICATORS

- Trauma to the head

IMMEDIATE ACTIONS

- Immobilize the neck.
- Make victim comfortable.

If unconscious, place victim on side.

CHECK & ACT

- **If bleeding from ear or nose without nose trauma:**
  - Suspect skull fracture and call **PAN-PAN** for medical advice.

    See 7. Emergency Communications, p. 37. ***(Action Guide)***
- **If unconscious or confused:**
  - Call **PAN-PAN** for medical advice and consider evacuation.
- **If conscious, alert, and oriented to time and place:**
  - Check extremities for movement and sensation.
- **If not able to fully move extremities or feel touch, suspect spinal injury:**
  - Call **MAYDAY** for evacuation

- **If able to fully move and feel touch**, suspect possible concussion: Check every 2 hours for:
  - Change in alertness, drowsiness, confusion
  - Difficulty with speech.
  - Unequal pupils
  - Asymmetrical grip or inability to move extremities.
  - Worsening headache.
  - If deterioration occurs, call **MAYDAY** for evacuation.
  - If no impairment after 24 hours, emergency is over.

Continued On Next Page

CHEST PAIN/HEART ATTACK

INDICATORS

- Chest pain without major trauma

IMMEDIATE ACTIONS

Get out of the elements, and make victim comfortable and warm.

CHECK & ACT

Determine:

- History of heart disease, heart burn, or similar chest pains
- Medications used by the person for these problems
- Location and radiation of pain
- Description and severity
- Inciting event
- What makes it better or worse

The three most common possibilities are:

1 If pain is associated with an isolated physical event, or is localized and made worse or better by movement or body position, it is likely from muscle or bone:
   - Immobilize or rest.
   - Use ibuprofen.
   - Use narcotics, if severe.

2 If pain is beneath the breast bone or in the upper stomach, is associated with recent food or alcohol, and is relieved by an antacid, it is likely from heartburn:
   - Use antacid for immediate relief.
   - Begin acid-reducing medication (omeprazole or ranitidine or Pepto-Bismol*) *Note: Pepto-Bismol may cause black tongue and black stools.
   - Avoid alcohol, coffee, chocolate, orange juice, and tomato sauces.

Continued On Next Page

3 If pain is severe, is beneath the breastbone, and is in or radiates to the left neck, shoulder, or arm, it suggests heart attack:

a) Other indicators include pallor, sweating, anxiety, sense of doom, nausea, rapid or irregular pulse, shallow, fast breathing.

b) Have person immediately chew a 325 milligram aspirin.

c) If the victim has a history of angina heart disease and has nitroglycerin, place under tongue one every three minutes for three doses. If not relieved, do not repeat.

d) Transmit PAN-PAN, and "I require medical advice"
See 7. Emergency Communications, p. 37. ***(Action Guide)***

e) If pain persists for more than 15 minutes, presume a heart attack.

f) Transmit **MAYDAY** and prepare to evacuate.

g) If Automatic Electronic Defibrillator (AED) is available, connect leads and follow directions.

INJURY TO LIMB

INDICATORS: BLEEDING

- Bleeding of upper or lower extremity

IMMEDIATE ACTIONS

1. Apply direct pressure to the wound, which almost always stops the bleeding
   - Initially use palm, and clean towel or cloth.
   - Then use sterile injury pad with direct pressure.
   - Elevate the injured limb.
2. If bleeding persists, DO NOT remove the sterile pad or dressing, but add additional dressings and pressure.
3. If necessary, apply a pressure bandage using an elastic wrap or a self-adherent wrap.
4. If swelling occurs near the bandage, or there is numbness, pins and needles sensation, or white or purplish skin color, reduce pressure.

CHECK & ACT

1. If bleeding persists, add pressure on arterial pressure point between the injury and the heart.
2. Call **PAN-PAN** for medical advice.

   See 7. Emergency Communications, p. 37. ***(Action Guide)***
3. Tourniquets are strongly discouraged and used as a last resort, and only with medical advice.
4. Call **MAYDAY** for evacuation.
5. Once a tourniquet is applied, DO NOT loosen or remove without medical advice.
6. Observe for signs of shock: rapid shallow breathing, pallor, sweating, cold extremities, confusion, restlessness, thready pulse, low blood pressure.

Continued On Next Page

INDICATORS: BROKEN LIMB

- Strong blow or fall on an extremity
- Pain in use or when bearing weight

IMMEDIATE ACTIONS

- **Immobilize** with a splint.
- Give pain relief medication.

CHECK & ACT

1. Check for danger signs:
   - Misalignment of the limb.
   - Visible bone.
   - Inability to move the extremity in its full range.
   - Loss of sensation distant from the injury.
   - Pallor or bluish color distant from the injury.
2. If any of above are present, call **PAN-PAN** and prepare for evacuation.

   See 7. Emergency Communications, p. 37. ***(Action Guide)***
3. If no danger signs are present, it may represent a bruise or an aligned fracture.
   - Continue splinting.
   - Observe for developing danger signs.
   - Gradually have person resume use of limb.

INJURY TO TRUNK

INDICATORS

- Hard blow or fall to the body that may result in internal organ damage and bleeding

IMMEDIATE ACTIONS

Place person in comfortable position, and keep warm and dry.

CHECK & ACT

1 Look for signs of internal bleeding.
   - Vomiting of blood or coffee ground–like material.
   - Coughing up blood or bloody froth.
   - Bloody or black tar-like stools.
   - Rigid, painful abdomen.
   - Pain with breathing, shortness of breath.
   - Weak pulse, blood pressure less than 100 systolic.
   - Light-headedness, confusion, restlessness, anxiety.

2 Check for pulse and breathing, and begin CPR if either is absent.

3 If any of the above signs are present, call **PAN PAN** and seek medical advice.

See 7. Emergency Communications, p. 37. ***(Action Guide)***

4 If none of the above signs are present, keep person comfortable and recheck every 2 hours until recovered.

CONFUSION/LETHARGY

INDICATORS

- Gradual onset of loss of judgment, ability to follow instructions, loss of interest, or slurred speech

HYPOTHERMIA

- Person shows mental confusion, inability to walk or perform physical tasks; typically after immersion or exposure to severe cold or wet conditions.
- Oral body temperature is <95 degrees F or <35 degrees C.
- Other signs include shivering or inability to talk coherently.

IMMEDIATE ACTIONS

- Remove from elements to a warm area.
- Remove wet clothing and dress in dry, warm clothing.
- Wrap in dry blanket or metallic warming blanket.
- Encourage drinking warm liquids; DO NOT administer alcoholic beverages.
- Apply hot water bottles to armpits and groin.
- If person is very confused, unable to cooperate, and not responding, call **PAN-PAN**, obtain medical advice and consider evacuation.

See 7. Emergency Communications, p. 37. ***(Action Guide)***

Continued On Next Page

HEAT STROKE

Heat exhaustion and heat stroke are caused by prolonged exposure to extreme heat. Each may be more likely in humid conditions, or with prolonged exertion and low consumption of water.

- Early symptoms are heat cramps, heavy sweating, nausea, feeling faint.
- Progressive symptoms include absence of sweating, hot, dry skin, body temperature >104 degrees F, or >40 degrees C.
- More severe symptoms include confusion, disorientation, diminishing consciousness.

IMMEDIATE ACTIONS

1 Shelter victim from heat.
2 Encourage fluid intake early but do not overhydrate
3 Initiate emergency cooling:
   - Remove excess clothing.
   - Immerse victim in cool water, or cover with water-soaked clothing or towels.
   - Give sips of cool water for core body cooling.
   - In severe situations, if possible, apply ice around neck, armpits, flanks, and groin.
4 For more severe symptoms, seek medical advice.
   See 7. Emergency Communications, p. 37. ***(Action Guide)***

Continued On Next Page

SEASICKNESS

Person is vomiting and unable to keep liquids and foods in stomach due to vessel motion, resulting in dehydration.

IMMEDIATE ACTIONS

- The seasick person should be offered options that do not interfere with vessel operations, such as resting below and in general staying out of the way as they cope.
- The person should avoid strong odors, such as diesel and waste.
- Keep the individual warm and dry.
- Medications are less effective after the onset of seasickness, so susceptible individuals should start them 24 hours before voyage.
- Medication should be tried before sail including: transdermal scopolamine, cinnarizine (Stugeron), diphenhyrdramine (Benadryl).
- Prolonged seasickness may lead to severe dehydration, confusion, and lethargy
- If this occurs, seek medical advice.

Continued On Next Page

ALLERGIC REACTIONS & STINGS

Allergic reactions are either localized or are generally not life-threatening, or are generalized involving the whole body and may be life-threatening.

Stabilize: Remove the causative agent.

ALLERGIC REACTION

INDICATORS

- Extensive hives, itching
- Swelling of eyelids, lips, tongue
- Difficulty breathing, tightness of the throat
- Pallor, thready pulse

IMMEDIATE ACTIONS

Determine the following through interview, if possible:

- History of precipitating event (food, etc).
- Prior similar episode(s).
- Personal medications available.

CHECK & ACT

1. Administer adrenalin injection (Ana-Kit, EpiPen) if competent administrator and injection are available.
2. Administer an antihistamine by mouth (chlorpheniramine in Ana-Kit, or diphenhydramine or others).
3. Repeat adrenalin in 30-60 minutes if symptoms return.
4. Repeat antihistamine in 2-4 hours if symptoms persist or return.

Continued On Next Page

MARINE-LIFE STINGS

IMMEDIATE ACTIONS

Determine the following through interview, if possible:

- History of precipitating event (sting, etc.).
- Prior similar episode(s).
- Personal medications available.

CHECK & ACT

1 If insect sting, remove stinger, if visible
  - Apply ice pack or cooling for 30 minutes for pain relief.
  - Use ibuprofen, or acetaminophen for pain relief as necessary.
  - If swelling occurs, use antihistamine (chlorpheniramine, diphenhydramine, or other).

2 If marine sting, remove tentacles or debris **without touching with bare hands**.
  - Wash with copious amounts of salt water.
  - Do NOT use vinegar, meat tenderizer or urine, because in some stings this may release additional toxins.
  - Scrape area with credit card or shave with shaving cream and razor to remove remaining stinging cells.
  - Pain relief, as necessary, with ibuprofen, acetaminophen.

9. Man Overboard

Utmost effort should be directed to avoid a man overboard situation. Have firm procedures for the use of life vests, harnesses, tethers, and jacklines to prevent MOB. Insist the crew clip-on when on deck or alone in the cockpit.

Train crew in the procedure you will use to recover a MOB.

If you become a MOB: hail, flash light, activate personal Emergency Position-Indicating Radio Beam (EPIRB) to alert the rest of the crew, swim only to recover a floatable aid, do not shed clothes, and do your best to preserve energy and heat by assuming a fetal position.

9

MOB Seen in Water ↓

MOB Not Seen ↓

MOB SEEN IN THE WATER

IMMEDIATE ACTIONS

1 **Maintain eye contact, point to the MOB.**
2 **Press MOB button** on GPS.
3 **Release MOB gear** (dan buoy; life/ring buoy; strobe light; drogue anchor); throw **floatable aids.**
4 **Alert all crew** to MOB.
5 **If there are complications or delays, transmit Mayday.**

RETURN TO MOB

- On a **small maneuverable boat**, stop in place, steer to avoid propellers touching MOB, and return to MOB directly.
- On a **larger boat**, with the MOB still visible, perform a single, round turn that will bring you back to the MOB in a circle.
- For still **larger vessels**, return to the MOB by executing a Racetrack Turn.

Continued On Next Page

RECOVERY

Approach

1 Keep MOB to leeward.
2 Prepare recovery gear and brief crew on your plan.
3 Approach MOB with steering speed, then drift on final approach.
4 Make direct contact or deploy lifesling.

Recovery

1 Use swimming platform if the sea permits, otherwise recover from amidship.
2 Consider deploying a dinghy.
3 To hoist MOB on board, use a block and tackle connected to upper deck or a boom.

Disabled MOB

- Deploy a swimmer to assist.
- Attach a stretcher made from a floorboard or cushions to assist MOB recovery.

MOB BACK ON BOARD

1 Assess MOB condition, administer first aid, if needed.
See 8. Medical Emergency, p. 47. ***(Action Guide)***
2 Verify all lines and equipment are out of the water before engaging the engine.
3 Cancel or restate **Mayday.**
See 7. Emergency Communications, p. 37. ***(Action Guide)***

MOB NOT SEEN

IMMEDIATE ACTIONS

1 **Release MOG gear** (Dan buoy, lifebuoy, strobe, and drogue)
2 **Press MOB button** on GPS.
3 **Note last course and speed.**
4 **Initiate the Williamson Turn** (turn full rudder to port until you motor 60 degrees off the original course; then turn full rudder to starboard until returning to reciprocal course on the original truck). Or use another turn to bring you to a reciprocal course from the MOB/GPS position.
5 **Debrief crew** where the MOB was last seen and establish best estimate of where and when the MOB event occurred.
6 Transmit **Mayday** to request assistance and coordinate systematic search.
See 7. Emergency Communications, p. 37. ***(Action Guide)***
7 Turn the boat to reciprocal course.

SEARCH

1 **Retrace** route, taking into account leeway and current.
2 **Use plotter to mark estimated location** of event and use it to plan and execute the **search between current position and last MOB seen position.**
3 **Assign all hands** to observation sectors with observation aids.
4 **If MOB still not found**, **initiate an expanded search pattern** based on current and wind conditions.

Continued On Next Page

RECOVERY

Approach

1 Keep MOB to leeward.
2 Prepare recovery gear and brief crew on your plan.
3 Approach MOB with steering speed, and drift to him with engine in neutral.
4 Make direct contact or deploy lifesling.

Recovery

1 Use swimming platform if the sea permits, otherwise recover from amidship.
2 Consider deploying a dinghy.
3 To hoist MOB on board, consider:
   - Lifesling connected to a block and tackle attached to top deck or to a boom.
   - Loop line connected to a winch or anchor windlass.

Disabled MOB, consider:

- Deploying a swimmer to assist.
- Attaching a stretcher made from a floorboard or cushions to assist MOB recovery.

MOB BACK ON BOARD

1 Assess MOB condition, administer first aid, if needed.
   See 8. Medical Emergency, p. 47. ***(Action Guide)***
2 Verify all lines and equipment are out of the water before engaging the engine.
3 Cancel or restate **Mayday.**
   See 7. Emergency Communications, p. 37. ***(Action Guide)***

10. Extreme Weather

With good weather forecasting, you can avoid most extreme weather, but not all. When sailing over a long distance and a long season, you should be prepared to encounter rough weather.

INDICATORS

a) Forecasts

b) Local observation:

- Barometric pressure
- Wind, strength and direction
- Waves, height and direction
- Clouds

At Dock ↓ | **At Anchor** ↓ | **At Sea** ↓

AT DOCK

CHECK & ACT

1 In safe harbor: don't depart.
2 Consider changing location within harbor.
3 Double your mooring lines.
4 Use additional chafing gear and fenders.
5 Assess potential risk from adjacent boats and take appropriate measures.
6 Consider using breast anchor(s) to avoid hitting the dock.

AT ANCHOR

CHECK & ACT

In safe anchorage, don't depart.

Consider:

1. The safety of your anchorage—whether it provides adequate protection and holding for the developing conditions.
2. Your boat's location within the anchorage.
3. The number and arrangement of your anchor(s).
4. The length of the anchor rode.
5. The risk from adjacent boats.
6. Using a snubber or steadying sail.
7. Chafing gear for anchor rode.
8. Reducing windage by folding the bimini and dodger and stowing superfluous items on deck.

Note: Before extreme conditions such as a tropical storm, move all items from deck and **get off the boat**.

AT SEA

Managing a boat in extreme weather is largely a problem of dealing with the **kinetic energy of waves.**

Large waves require **active boat handling**, using rudder, engine maneuvers, and tabs to avoid breaching and rollover. This is difficult in daylight and even harder at night.

Execute extreme weather checklist.

See 5. Heavy Weather Preparation, p. 21. ***(Safety Checklist)***

- **If able to reach safe harbor, do so, considering:**
  - Ease of entrance to the harbor.
  - Lee shore en route.
  - Space inside the harbor.

  Note: Radio your intentions to harbor master and Coast Guard.

- **If unable to reach safe harbor:**
  - Head offshore to gain sea room.
  - Maneuver away from storm center.

IN A STORM

- **When able to motor in a desired direction:**
  - **Motor to windward:** Steer diagonally into approaching waves, steer directly into the crest when it is approaching, and then fall off to your desired direction as you descend the wave. .
  - **With the sea on the beam:** When a breaking crest approaches, change the boat direction to present your bow to the crest and then resume your course.

Continued On Next Page

- **When motoring downwind:** Use the engine and the rudder to maintain a position on the **back of a wave**, avoiding breaking waves into the boat's exposed aft deck.

If keeping course is too difficult:

- **Motor downwind:** Maintain a position **on the back of a wave.** If you can take the waves on your aft deck, slow down and stabilize your direction by streaming lines or drogues from behind.
- **When no sea room:**
  - Deploy a sea anchor or a drogue.
  - Use the engine to keep your bow to the sea, using minimal speed to hold your position.
  - If being pushed toward danger, when depth permits, consider anchoring on the longest rode.

Note: If likely to be swept on lee shore or flouder, transmit **Mayday** early to allow for timely rescue.

See 7. Emergency Communications, p. 37. ***(Action Guide)***

Continued On Next Page

TROPICAL STORM

Tropical storms are best avoided by paying close attention to tropical storm seasonal patterns and forecasts.

If you are caught in a storm, plot the storm's center and its path.

In the northern hemisphere, the storm's dangerous semicircle is on the right side of its path.

- **To escape the dangerous semicircle, motor 90 degrees away from the storm truck.** Be careful not to cross the storm's path. However, if your boat speed and disntance from the storm center permit, consider crossing in navigable semicircle long before the center arrives.
- In the **navigable semicircle**, motor down wind and away from the storm center.
- Monitor your position in relation to the storm center by facing the wind. The center is on your right hand side and a bit behind.

In the southern hemisphere, the dangerous and the navigable semicircles are reversed, as are the directions of escape.

Extra tropical storms, some of hurricane strength, form in higher latitudes. These storms require similar strategies of escape. **Extra tropical storms cover larger areas, move fast, and have the added complication of frontal passages, which makes for a messy sea.**

11. Abandon Ship

Do not abandon ship as long as it is afloat. It is a better platform than a life raft to survive on and is easier for rescuers to find.

INDICATORS

The boat is about to sink

IMMEDIATE ACTION

1 Order crew to **prepare** to abandon ship—make sure the order is conveyed and understood by all.
2 All crew members should don life jackets and warm clothes, and have personal documents, medications, credit cards, etc.
3 Allocate crew duties and responsibilities.
4 **Transmit Mayday.**
See 7. Emergency Communications, p. 37. ***(Action Guide)***
5 Communicate your position, nature of distress, number of people, injuries. Keep communication engaged. Do not switch channels or radios.
6 Activate EPIRB.
7 Consider alerting your "on-shore advocate" and keep him/her on standby.

11

Continued On Next Page

Abandon Ship

CHECK & ACT

1 Prepare to launch life raft and dinghy with its pumps and repair kit, and check outboard and fuel for dinghy
2 Prepare the ditch bag and any additional equipment to take with you:
   - EPIRB
   - Handheld VHF, mobile phone, and satellite phone
   - Flares
   - Compass and charts
   - Portable GPS
   - Flashlights
   - First aid kit
   - Knives
   - Emergency water
   - Emergency food
   - Space blankets and warm clothing
   - Ship documents

   If you have time, take more food and water.

ABANDON SHIP

1 Deploy life raft and launch dinghy. Connect them with a short line.
2 Board agile people first and last.
3 **Account for all crew** and cut loose.

WARNING!
Do not inflate the raft prematurely. In extreme weather, it will be difficult to keep the life raft and the dinghy tethered to the boat for long.

12. Rescue

The legal and moral responsibility to save lives at sea is universally recognized. Your decision to transmit a **Mayday** will trigger life-threatening actions by others. Consider it seriously.

INDICATORS

- Life-threatening situation
- Boat at risk
- Boat sinking

IMMEDIATE ACTIONS

1 Transmit **Mayday**.

See 7. Emergency Communications, p. 37. ***(Action Guide)***

2 Verify that communication is established and do not change radios or channels. If unsuccessful, use all other means of communication.

3 Activate EPIRB.

4 Be prepared to communicate:

- Your GPS location and/or distance and bearing from a known landmark.
- Individual rescue or full crew and number of crew on board.
- Injuries.
- Boat condition and identifying details.

5 Prepare pyrotechnics for immediate use.

Continued On Next Page

Ship Rescue

Helicopter Rescue

FULL CREW RESCUE

Prepare to take:

- Boat documents.
- Personal papers, passports, money, credit cards.
- Valuables.

INDIVIDUAL RESCUE

Prepare to accompany individual with:

- Medical history and information relevant to the injury.
- Personal papers.

SHIP RESCUE

1 When you see a rescue vessel but it doesn't see you, or upon the vessel's instruction, operate pyrotechnics.
   - Daylight: smoke, flares.
   - Night: torch, flares, deck light, and all other navigation lights.
2 Ask ship to position you in the lee and use its rigid inflatable to approach you.
3 Prepare long lines and fenders to use when transferring people to boat or ship.

WARNING!
Assume major damage to your boat and rig if forced to approach alongside ship in any seaway.

HELICOPTER RESCUE

1. **Brief the crew** before the helicopter arrives as communication will be difficult once it is overhead.
2. Be prepared to **obey the helicopter crew** or the swimmer's instructions.
3. Limit your radio contact with the helicopter to necessary responses only.
4. Clear the hoist area, usually port side aft, of anything loose.

UPON APPROACH

- **Under power**, proceed in the direction and speed given by the helicopter pilot, usually with the wind twenty degrees off the port bow.
- **At night**, illuminate the deck but avoid shining lights or laser at the helicopter.
- Pickup will be done as instructed by the helicopter, usually from the deck or, in rough seas, from a towed dinghy, life raft, or directly from the water.
- When cable is lowered:
  - a) Do not touch cable until it is grounded
  - b) Do not attach the cable or the hoist to the boat or let them snag on anything.

13. Skipper Disabled

It is the responsibility of the skipper to prepare the crew for the possibility of becoming incapacitated. The skipper should assign crew responsibilities and practice for such a contingency.

Members of the crew need basic proficiency in:

- Starting and stopping the engine.
- Disengaging and engaging the autopilot.
- Using the VHF and other communication equipment.
- Anchoring.
- Using basic safety equipment.

Skipper Overboard ↓

Skipper Injured ↓

SKIPPER OVERBOARD

IMMEDIATE ACTIONS

1 Keep eye contact and point to MOB.
2 Throw floatation aids.
3 Stop the boat:
   a) Put engine in neutral.
   b) Disconnect autopilot.
4 Press MOB button on the GPS.
5 If capable, deploy lifesling, approach MOB, and recover.
   See 9. Man Overboard, p. 67. ***(Action Guide)***

ASK FOR HELP

1 Transmit **Mayday** and seek outside help and advice.
   See 7. Emergency Communications, p. 37. ***(Action Guide)***
2 Use all communication equipment available—VHF, SSB, satellite phone, mobile phone, voice.
3 Proceed to recover with whatever help is available.

SKIPPER INJURED

IMMEDIATE ACTIONS

- **If the boat is motoring into immediate danger:**
  Stop the boat.
  1 Put the engine in neutral.
  2 Disconnect autopilot.

- **If the boat is not in immediate danger:**
  Continue motoring and do not maneuver

- **If the skipper is in immediate danger:**
  Administer first aid *See 8. Medical Emergency, p. 47.* ***(Action Guide)***

- **If the skipper is not in immediate danger:**
  Assess the situation before calling for help. You have time to consider your options and what you need.

ASK FOR HELP

1 Transmit **Mayday** and seek outside help and advice.
See 7. Emergency Communications, p. 37. ***(Action Guide)***
2 Use all communication equipment available—VHF, SSB, satellite phone, mobile phone, voice.